Venous
Thromboembolism

For Dr Keith Leiper who always encouraged books – thank you for teaching me about being a doctor. And for John – for being ginger. And because I promised.

Venous Thromboembolism
A Nurse's Guide to Prevention and Management

Dr Ellen Welch MBChB, MCEM, BA (Hons) Medical Journalism
Ski Field Doctor, Core medical, Queenstown Medical Centre, New Zealand

With contribution from

Lynda Bonner RGN, DipHE Nursing
Coagulation Nurse Specialist, King's College Hospital, London

⊛WILEY-BLACKWELL

A John Wiley & Sons, Ltd., Publication

This edition first published 2010
© 2010 John Wiley & Sons, Ltd.

Wiley-Blackwell is an imprint of John Wiley & Sons, formed by the merger of Wiley's global Scientific, Technical and Medical business with Blackwell Publishing.

Registered office
John Wiley & Sons Ltd, The Atrium, Southern Gate, Chichester, West Sussex, PO19 8SQ, United Kingdom

Editorial office
John Wiley & Sons Ltd, The Atrium, Southern Gate, Chichester, West Sussex, PO19 8SQ, United Kingdom

For details of our global editorial offices, for customer services and for information about how to apply for permission to reuse the copyright material in this book please see our website at www.wiley.com/wiley-blackwell.

The right of the author to be identified as the author of this work has been asserted in accordance with the Copyright, Designs and Patents Act 1988.

Wiley also publishes its books in a variety of electronic formats. Some content that appears in print may not be available in electronic books.

Designations used by companies to distinguish their products are often claimed as trademarks. All brand names and product names used in this book are trade names, service marks, trademarks or registered trademarks of their respective owners. The publisher is not associated with any product or vendor mentioned in this book. This publication is designed to provide accurate and authoritative information in regard to the subject matter covered. It is sold on the understanding that the publisher is not engaged in rendering professional services. If professional advice or other expert assistance is required, the services of a competent professional should be sought.

Library of Congress Cataloging-in-Publication Data

Welch, Ellen.
    Venous thromboembolism : a nurses guide to prevention and management / Ellen Welch ; with contribution from Lynda Bonner.
        p. ; cm.
    Includes bibliographical references and index.
    ISBN 978-0-470-51189-3 (pbk.)
    1. Thromboembolism–Nursing.   I. Bonner, Lynda.   II. Title.
    [DNLM: 1. Venous Thromboembolism–nursing.   WY 152.5 W439v 2010]
    RC694.3.W45 2010
    616.1′450231–dc22

                                                                    2009038801

A catalogue record for this book is available from the British Library.

Set in 10 on 12 pt Palatino by Toppan Best-set Premedia Limited
Printed and bound in Singapore by Fabulous Printers Pte Ltd

1 2010

Contents

Contributors

Dr Ellen Welch
MBChB, MCEM, BA (Hons) Medical Journalism
Ellen Welch qualified from the University of Liverpool in 2004 and since then has worked in a variety of settings around the world, with the majority of her experience based in a medical and emergency medicine environment. She has worked as a cruise ship physician in the Caribbean and a ski field doctor in New Zealand and undertook the majority of her emergency medicine training in Leeds. Her interest in medical journalism has led to several publications in nursing and medical journals.

Lynda Bonner
RGN, DipHE Nursing
Lynda qualified in 1992 as an RGN from Royal Victoria Hospital, Belfast and has worked within coagulation and thrombosis at Kings College Hospital since 2002.
She currently leads a team of six coagulation nurse specialists at the King's thrombosis centre, providing leadership in the promotion and delivery of evidence-based nursing care for patients who are at risk of, or who have developed venous thromboembolism. The team, plays a leading role in the prevention, diagnosis and treatment of VTE, and in anticoagulation management.
Lynda has completed modules on Evidence Based Practice at Degree level and modules on Leadership and Project Management at Masters level.

Preface

Venous thromboembolism (VTE) received a flurry of media attention early in 2005 after the House of Commons Select Committee for Health published a critical report on the subject. According to the report, 25 000 patients in England die each year from VTE, which is more than the combined total of deaths from breast cancer, AIDS and road traffic injuries.

What is perhaps more alarming than this figure in itself is the fact that many of these deaths are preventable. By recognizing high-risk patients and starting them on what have been proven to be safe and cost-effective prophylactic treatments, lives can be saved.

Since 2005, many organizations have been working hard to promote the issue among both the public and health professionals. Dedicated thrombosis teams have been established in many hospitals throughout the UK, and VTE risk assessments upon admission to hospital have become mandatory. Follow-up audits by the Department of Health show some improvement in the use of thromboprophylaxis, but there remains room for improvement. The National Institute of Clinical Excellence was commissioned to address this problem and a report on reducing the risk of VTE in surgical inpatients was published in 2007. Similar guidelines for patients admitted to hospital are expected in early 2010, followed by guidelines on management of VTE in 2012.

In the meantime, since VTE is a condition that can affect patients presenting to all specialty areas, it is important that health professionals can recognize patients at risk and implement prophylaxis. This book aims to act as a comprehensive resource for nurses and other health care professionals who seek for a greater understanding of the condition. It hopes to provide practical tips and theoretical knowledge to enable nurses to deliver informed quality care to their patients.

Ellen Welch
April 2009

Acknowledgements

Thanks to Dr Tom Kennedy at the Royal Liverpool University Hospital, who first enlightened me about the issue of VTE. Thanks to Dr Robin Illingworth at St James's University Hospital, Leeds, for his encouragement, and thanks also to the Leeds teaching Hospitals Trust for the use of their CDU protocols. To the team aboard the Carnival Freedom – I'm grateful I was given the time to work on the manuscript and a special thank you to Dr Melissa Perry for allowing me to do the research. Finally, big thanks to Steve and Levente, whose harassment and support helped me to finish this book ... eventually.

Ellen Welch

With sincere thanks to: Dr Aidan McManus and Lucy Hyatt (MMRX Communications); Dr Arya, Dr Patel, Emma Coker, Lindsey Wood (Kings College Hospital); AMTEC Consulting plc, ArjoHuntleigh Group, and Covidien (Industry); Tim Dumbledon (CEP); Shalni Gulati and Angela Monaghan (City University, London) for their various contributions towards this chapter. I would also like to express my thanks to the excellent Thrombosis Team and Senior Management Team at Kings College Hospital, who ensured that usual service for patients continued whilst allowing dedicated time for this chapter to be written.

Lynda Bonner

What is VTE?

Overview

This chapter covers the basics of VTE, opening with some defini-
tions and statistics from the literature to illustrate the size of the
problem. Recurrent VTE and idiopathic VTE are discussed and
the importance of prevention is highlighted. The economic burden
of VTE in the United Kingdom is discussed and comparisons are
made globally. The changes in our understanding of VTE are
detailed in a chronological history of the condition, which places
our current understanding in context.

An introduction

Venous thromboembolism (VTE) is the term used to encompass the
two related conditions of deep vein thrombosis (DVT) and pulmonary
embolism (PE). Venous thrombosis is the term used to describe conditions in which blood clots (thrombi) form in a vein, causing partial or
complete obstruction to blood flow. The 'deep veins' of the calves,
thighs and pelvis are the most common sites of thrombus formation,
although clots can also form in more proximal veins and in the upper
extremities. Venous thrombosis of the 'deep veins' is known as DVT.

Venous Thromboembolism: A Nurses Guide to Prevention and Management   By Ellen Welch
© 2010 John Wiley & Sons, Ltd.

If a piece of the blood clots breaks off and travels from its site of formation through the venous system, it is known as an 'embolus' (from the
Greek *embolos*, meaning wedge or plug). If the clot is carried through
the blood stream, through the chambers of the heart and into the pulmonary circulation, it can become lodged in the arteries of the lungs,
where it is known as a PE. A large PE that restricts blood flow to the
lungs can be fatal (Chapter 2 provides further information on the
pathophysiology of the condition).

Each of the stages of VTE (i.e. calf DVT, proximal DVT, PE) may or
may not be associated with clinical symptoms, depending upon the
severity of the thrombosis, the adequacy of the collateral vessels (the
vessels surrounding the occluded vein) and the extent of the inflammation caused by the blockage. The general health of a patient is an
additional factor that can influence presentation. For example, a moderately sized PE may cause no symptoms in an otherwise healthy
patient, but may result in severe symptoms or even death on a background of advanced cardiopulmonary disease (Kearon 2003). Chapters
5 and 6 delve further into the clinical presentation of the two conditions
and the investigations and treatments currently used in practice.

Both symptomatic and asymptomatic VTE have been associated
with fatalities and acute morbidity. A report commissioned by the
House of Commons Health Committee in 2005 estimated that VTE in
hospitalized patients causes up to 32 000 deaths from PE per year in
the United Kingdom, as well as causing significant chronic health problems due to post-thrombotic limb and venous ulceration. Approximately 100 000 people in England and Wales suffer with venous leg
ulcers following a DVT, which are often resistant to treatment, leading
to prolonged hospitalization and discomfort to patients, costing the
NHS an estimated £100–300 million each year (Bosanquet 1992; Laing
1992). The total cost of managing VTE within the NHS is thought to be
£640 million each year (House of Commons Health Committee 2005).

Public awareness in the United Kingdom

The death of a 28 year-old woman from a PE after a long-haul flight
from Sydney to London in Autumn 2000 provoked a media frenzy
surrounding 'economy class syndrome' and 'traveller's thrombosis'.
However, the risks of hospital-acquired VTE remained unpublicized –
which is quite extraordinary, considering the impact the disease has on
national morbidity and mortality figures. Frustrated by this lack of
awareness, a group of health professionals founded Lifeblood, a thrombosis charity with the intention to increase awareness and research
funds for thrombosis (Hunt 2008).

In 2004, representatives from the charity met with the House of Commons Select Committee to highlight the issues. Emphasis was given to the fact that at least 50% of the deaths attributed to VTE were related to hospital admission, yet, despite the opportunity for these patients to receive thromboprophylaxis, it was not being implemented. It was pointed out that only 20% of eligible patients were receiving prophylaxis and health care professionals appeared ignorant of the risks (Hunt 2008).

The Chief Medical Officer agreed with the issues raised and wrote to all doctors in 2005, informing them of good practice guidelines regarding VTE prevention (House of Commons Health Committee 2005). It was then that the National Institute for Clinical Excellence was commissioned to produce thromboprophylaxis guidelines for all hospitalized patients, and a VTE Expert Working Group was established to report on how best practice could be promoted and implemented (Hunt 2008).

The expert working group recommended that all inpatients required a mandatory VTE risk assessment regarding their need for thromboprophylaxis, and that thrombosis teams should be established within hospitals to ensure that this is implemented (CMO 2007). National audits have been carried out annually by the All Party Parliamentary Thrombosis Group (APPTG) since these recommendations were made. The 2007 findings were disappointing and although 99% of trusts were aware of the guidelines, only 32% of them were undertaking a risk assessment for hospitalized patients (APPTG 2007). The Department of Health responded to this by publicizing a DVT Risk Assessment Tool in 2008 (see Appendix 1) and the follow-up audit carried out in the same year showed improvements. In 2008, 70% of acute NHS trusts declared that they were undertaking a documented VTE risk assessment in line with the recommendations of the Chief Medical Officer (APPTG 2008).

The feeling among many health professionals is that VTE is still more of a 'Cinderella issue' than it should be. The media thrive on stories concerning hospital-acquired infections, which account for about 6000 deaths each year in the United Kingdom, yet ignore hospital-acquired VTE – which causes significantly more. The charity Lifeblood have done much to increase public awareness in the United Kingdom; one such method was the institution of an annual 'National Thrombosis Week'; another was creating accessible information on the subject on the internet (Hunt 2008).

With increasing public awareness of VTE and government incentives mandating thromboprophylaxis in hospitals, it is hoped that future mortality figures attributable to VTE will be on the decline.

The scale of the problem

Determining the number of people who develop VTE each year has proved to be a challenge. Clinical symptoms are notoriously unreliable and the disease can often present 'silently', with no symptoms whatsoever (Verstraete 1997), meaning that many people may have VTE that has gone unrecognized. Conversely, a large number of cases of PE diagnosed at autopsy were included in the figures of some studies whether or not they were symptomatic, failing to take into account other pathology responsible for death and resulting in an overrepresentation in some of the data (White 2003). Despite these difficulties in determining exact incidence rates, it is clear that VTE remains a major public health problem and that concentrating on its prevention is key.

The incidence of VTE

A number of studies focusing on the epidemiology of the disease have been carried out worldwide, with the vast majority of the data being generated in the United States. A study over a 25 year period demonstrated that as many as 145 individuals per 100000 in the general population develop symptomatic DVT and up to 69 individuals per 100000 experience a PE (Silverstein 1998). More recent studies have suggested that the incidence of VTE is about 120 per 100000 people per year (Heit et al. 2001; Cushman et al. 2004). The higher figures cited by Silverstein are thought to reflect the large number of cases detected at autopsy. A review of several large American studies compiled by White (2003) suggest that the incidence of first-time symptomatic VTE, standardized for age and sex in predominantly Caucasian Americans, was in the range 71–117 cases per 100000 population. Based on this information, researchers have estimated that over 300000 United States citizens develop a first lifetime VTE each year (Heit 2005). Furthermore, recent computer modelling suggests that more than 900000 incident or recurrent, fatal and non-fatal VTE events occur in the United States annually, which is more than the estimated number of strokes ($n = 700000$) and heart attacks ($n = 865000$) (Heit et al. 2005). The incidence of VTE does not appear to have changed significantly over the last 25 years (Heit et al. 2006).

European studies have collected similar figures. A French study from 2001 found that new cases of DVT occur at a rate of about 87 per 100000 of the population, with PEs occurring at a rate of 46 per 100000 (Oger 2000). A Swedish study confirmed a DVT incidence of 117 per 100000 (Nordstrom et al. 1992). Lindblad et al. (1991) carried out a population-based autopsy study, which showed that autopsy-diagnosed fatal PE occurs in around 40 per 100000 population. Using this incidence-based approach, it is estimated that VTE has an incidence of 145 per 100000 diagnosed premortem and 47 per 100000 diagnosed at post mortem (House of Commons Health Committee 2005).

The VTE Impact Assessment Group in Europe (VITAE) used an epidemiological model developed by clinical and epidemiological thrombosis specialists working across Europe and the United States to derive estimates of total VTE events. The total annual burden of VTE in the 25 EU member states (population 454 million) was estimated to be 640000 symptomatic DVT and 383000 PE (Department of Health 2007).

In the United Kingdom this equates to approximately 59000 new cases of DVT and 29500 new cases of non-fatal PE per year (House of Commons Health Committee 2005). Initial treatment of VTE is costly and patients often go on to develop serious long-term complications which inevitably add to the cost burden on health services. Most patients with VTE require more than one diagnostic test, as well as a prolonged hospital stay involving treatment with heparin and multiple blood tests to monitor progress. The Office for Healthcare Economics estimated the annual cost in the United Kingdom of treating patients with postsurgical DVT and PE in 1993 was up to £222.8 million. The total cost to the United Kingdom for the management of VTE is estimated at £640 million. In addition to this, the long-term expenditure to care for those patients with chronic complications such as venous ulcers is thought to amount to £400 million (House of Commons Health Committee 2005).

Factors influencing the figures

Age
Incidence of VTE varies considerably, depending on an individual's age. In persons 15 years old or younger there are less than five cases per 100000 of the population annually. This figure rises exponentially with age to around 500 cases per 100000 of the population at age 80 years (Anderson *et al.* 1991; Silverstein 1998; White 2003). As the population ages, the number of deaths each year due to PE is also predicted to grow (Heit *et al.* 2005).

Sex
The use of oral contraceptives and hormone replacement therapy have been associated with VTE in women, but published data have shown no consistent differences in the incidence of VTE between the sexes (Nordstrom *et al.* 1992). Silverstein *et al.* (1998) noted a slightly higher incidence among women during childbearing years, but a higher rate

in men after the age of 50. The overall age-adjusted incidence rate was found to be 114 per 100 000 in men and 105 per 100 000 in women, with a male : female sex ratio of 1.2 : 1 (Heit 2008).

Race

Race has also been shown to effect incidence rates of VTE. Compared to Caucasians, studies have shown that African-Americans have an incidence of VTE approximately 30% higher, while Asian and Native American subjects show an incidence almost 70% lower (White *et al.* 1998 and 2003; Klatsky *et al.* 2000). An explanation for the lower incidence in Asian populations has not been found, but it has been suggested that it may relate to a lower prevalence of genetic factors predisposing to VTE, such as factor V Leiden. This condition, which causes hypercoagulability and a propensity to VTE, is described further in Chapter 5; it has been shown to have a 0.5% prevalence in Asian populations compared to 5% in Caucasians (Ridker *et al.* 1997; Gregg *et al.* 1997; Angchaisuksiri *et al.* 2000).

Season

The seasonal variation of VTE has been observed in various French studies. Bounameaux *et al.* (1996) found no relation to the incidence of DVT and time of year, but a large data set (*n* = 127 318) analysed by Boulay in 2001 discovered a 15% rise in VTE admissions during winter months and 15% fewer admissions during the summer. Further research is needed to confirm this finding, but it has been suggested that the figures are related to a decline in physical activity during the winter months, thus showing an inverse relationship between physical activity and the development of VTE (White 2003).

It is clear from the figures listed above that the presence of various risk factors, such as increasing age, have been shown to influence which patients develop VTE. In a community review of 1231 consecutive patients treated for VTE, 96% had at least one risk factor (Anderson *et al.* 1992) and risk appears to increase in proportion to the number of risk factors an individual has (Anderson *et al.* 2003). Specific risk factors and evidence for identifying which patients are at risk are discussed more comprehensively in Chapter 5.

Mortality rates

Estimates of mortality rates from VTE have varied widely among the studies that have been performed to date. VTE often affects patients with other concurrent diseases that reduce survival, such as cancer, which makes exact mortality figures difficult to establish. In the United States, it is estimated that 50 000–200 000 people die of PE each year

(Anderson 1995; Clagett *et al.* 1998; Dismuke *et al.* 1986; Horlander *et al.* 2003), which is thought to exceed the number of deaths due to myocardial infarction and stroke (Heit *et al.* 2005).

Survival after PE is much worse than after DVT alone (Douketis *et al.* 1998) – almost a quarter die suddenly and approximately 40% die within 3 months (Heit *et al.* 1999).

Some studies have shown that this mortality rate is decreasing (Horlander *et al.* 2003; Heit *et al.* 1999), while others state that it is stable (Goldhaber 1998). The mortality rate within 3 months of a venous thromboembolic event has been documented at 15–17.5% (Goldhaber 1997; Heit *et al.* 1999; Horlander *et al.* 2003). In individuals older than 65 years of age, Siddique *et al.* (1996) reported a fatality rate after diagnosis of PE of 16.1% in African-Americans and 12.9% in Caucasians. Data collected more recently by the RIETE registry (an ongoing, international, multicentre, prospective cohort of consecutive patients presenting with symptomatic VTE confirmed by objective testing) describe a three month mortality rate from fatal PE at 1.68%, with an overall mortality rate of 8.65%, and cite PE as a cause of death in 19.4% of patients in their study (Laporte *et al.* 2008).

In the United Kingdom it has been estimated that PE may account for rates of sudden death at up to 0.40 per 1000 population (Lindblad *et al.* 1991), equating to over 24000 deaths per year. A retrospective analysis of autopsy reports carried out in the 1980s found PE as a cause of death in 10% of general hospital patients (1% of all admissions) and 83% of these patients also had DVT in the legs at autopsy (Sandler *et al.* 1989). The VTE Impact Assessment Group in Europe (VITAE) estimated VTE-related deaths in Europe to be at 480000 annually. Of these deaths, 7% had been diagnosed with VTE and treated, 34% were estimated to be sudden fatal PE and 59% followed undetected PE (Department of Health 2007). The annual population death rate from VTE was about 0.1%, which in the United Kingdom, with a population of 60 million, equates to over 60000 deaths annually (Department of Health 2007).

Although the figures may vary, researchers are consistent about the clinical predictors that put patients at risk of fatal PE, and agree that identification of high-risk patients is important to adapt treatment to the level of risk (Laporte *et al.* 2008). The major clinical factors predictive of fatal PE in studies to date are advanced age, cancer, immobilization for neurological disease, systolic arterial hypotension, underlying cardiovascular disease and chronic lung or congestive heart failure (Laporte *et al.* 2008; Heit *et al.* 1999; Goldhaber *et al.* 1999). Numerous clinical trials over the past 30 years have shown that thromboprophylaxis reduces the frequency of VTE and thus deaths from fatal PE (see Chapter 6 for more information).

Recurrent VTE

VTE is a chronic disease, with about 30% of patients developing recurrence within the next 10 years (Heit *et al.* 2000; Schulman S *et al.* 2006). Recurrence appears to be highest within the first 6–12 months since the initial event (Heit 2008), with a recurrence rate of approximately 7% at 6 months (White 2003). Factors that appear to predict recurrence include male gender, increasing patient age and body mass index, neurological disease with lower limb paresis and active cancer (Heit *et al.* 2000; McRae *et al.* 2006). 'Idiopathic' VTE (VTE unassociated with surgery/trauma/identifiable underlying cause) is an independant predictor for recurrence in itself and those patients with thrombophilic tendancies are also at risk (Heit 2008). A possible link has been found with recurrent VTE and those patients with a persistently increased plasma fibrin D-dimer level (Palareti *et al.* 2006) and those with residual venous thrombosis (Prandoni *et al.* 2002).

Anticoagulation is effective at preventing recurrence, but the duration of anticoagulation does not seem to affect the risk of recurrence once primary therapy for the incident event is stopped (Schulman *et al.* 2006). After stopping anticoagulation therapy, the risk of recurrence for patients with transient risk factors, e.g. recent surgery, is approximately 3% per year, whereas in patients with a continuing risk factor, e.g. malignancy or idiopathic thrombosis, the risk is at least 10% per year (Kearon 2003).

Idiopathic VTE

Idiopathic VTE is defined as thrombosis that occurs in the absence of any identifiable risk factors. Approximately 50% of patients presenting with first idiopathic or juvenile VTE have an underlying thrombophilia (Anderson *et al.* 2003). Apparent idiopathic VTE is often found to have malignancy as its underlying cause and studies have shown a 5% incidence of previously undiagnosed cancer in patients presenting with VTE (Baron *et al.* 1998). Patients with idiopathic thrombosis have a high risk of experiencing a recurrent event and indefinite-duration anticoagulation therapy is advocated in such patients (Goldhaber 2004).

A timeline of our understanding

Our understanding of venous disease has been accumulating for well over 2000 years. Advances in related areas have also contributed towards what we know today. What follows is a chronological record of the discoveries that have provided us with a greater appreciation of venous thromboembolic disease today.

Despite its frequency today, there is little specific reference to venous thrombosis in antiquity. In artwork from ancient Egypt, Greece, Rome, Persia and South America there are representations of varicose veins and ulcers but very little suggestive of VTE.

2650–1550 BC

The first reference to peripheral venous disease was recorded in on one of the oldest preserved medical documents, the Ancient Egyptian Ebers papyrus (1550 BC) and documented the potential 'fatal haemorrhage' that may ensue from surgery on 'serpentine windings' or varicose veins. The Chinese physician Huang Ti described pathological haemostasis earlier still, in 2650 BC, writing: 'when the blood coagulates within the foot it causes pain and chills' – but this could of course be referring to arterial thrombosis (Dickson 2004).

460–377 BC

Hippocrates (460–377 BC) made many references to the vascular system and ulcers and was first to use the term 'leucophlegmasia' to describe bilateral leg oedema, most likely due to conditions such as heart failure and liver cirrhosis but possibly also due to post-thrombotic oedema (Anning 1957). He observed the magical transformation of blood from liquid into a solid and reasoned that it was due to cooling.

AD 129–200

The Greek physician Galen (AD 129–200) also recognized this phenomenon and introduced the term 'thrombosis', which is Greek for curdling. Galen was also first to describe the four classic symptoms of inflammation (redness, pain, heat and swelling). Early physicians from Hippocrates onwards followed the Theory of Humours, which taught that the body is made up of four 'humours' (blood, phlegm, black bile and yellow bile). An imbalance of these humours was thought to be the cause of all diseases, and practices of blood letting and placing hot cups on patients were done in an effort to redress this balance. Humouralism was widely practised until the late nineteenth century, when it was decisively displaced by Rudolf Virchow's theories of cellular pathology (see Box 1.1).

Box 1.1 Rudolf Ludwig Karl Virchow

Born in October 1821 in Schievelbein, eastern Pomerania (today's Poland), as the only son of a merchant, Rudolf Virchow (Figure 1.1) is considered by many to have been the most prominent German physician of the nineteenth century (Safavi-Abbasi *et al.* 2006).

Describing him as an overachiever would be something of an understatement. Among numerous accomplishments, he pioneered the modern concept of 'cell theory' to explain the effects of disease in organisms at a cellular level, displacing the long-held belief that disease was caused by an imbalance of the four 'humours'. He recognized the blood-borne pathogenesis of syphilis and was the first to describe leukaemia (Safavi-Abbasi *et al.* 2006). His name has also become eponymous with an enlarged left supraclavicular node, 'Virchow's node', which is indicative of gastrointestinal malignancy.

Virchow's 'epoch-making' paper on embolism was published in 1847, popularizing the terms 'thrombosis' and 'embolism' to describe clots or 'curds' in blood vessels. He observed: '... the

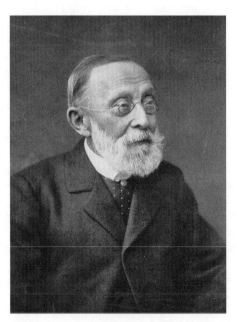

Figure 1.1 Rudolf Ludwig Karl Virchow. Courtesy of the Clendening History of Medicine Library, University of Kansas Medical Center.

detachment of fragments from the end of the softening thrombus which are carried along by the current of blood and driven into remote vessels. This gives rise to the very frequent process on which I have bestowed the name of Embolia' (Virchow 1978).

Although Virchow's name is now eponymous with the triad of predisposing factors to VTE (irregularity of the vessel lumen, impaired blood flow and increased coagulability), the literature suggests that the three elements had been established as a cause prior to the work of Virchow and he never laid claim to these observations. The term 'Virchow's triad' did not come into use until the 1950s (Anning 1957) and its components were not fully agreed on in the literature until the 1930s (Dickson 2004). Regardless of its origins, the term still remains clinically relevant today.

Virchow acted as a political revolutionary throughout his life, upholding his belief that 'the physician is the natural advocate for the poor' (Pearce 2002). He promoted public health issues such as sewage disposal, hospital design, public hygiene and meat inspection and incidentally also discovered trichinosis (Safavi-Abbasi *et al.* 2006)

His provocative ideas were viewed with some hostility among his peers, and various medical journals refused to publish some of his work. Undeterred by this, he founded his own medical journal together with the pathologist Benno Ernst Heinrich Reinhardt. He was a keen anthropologist and contributed to the development of anthropology as a modern science. He continued to lecture, write, edit, research and serve in political bodies until his death.

Virchow died in 1902 at the age of 81, when, still active and energetic, he jumped prematurely from a moving passenger tram in Berlin. He fractured his hip and died soon afterwards in hospital. He led an immensely productive life, making monumental contributions to medical sciences. An exhaustive list of his publications and biographies can be found in Ole Daniel Enerson (http://www.whonamedit.com/doctor.cfm/912.html) (Safavi-Abbasi *et al.* 2006).

1271

The earliest documented case of venous thrombosis comes from an illustrated manuscript presented to the Cardinal of Bourbonnoys in the fifteenth century and outlines an account of a man suffering with classic symptoms in 1271 (Dexter *et al.* 1974). Reports that accumulated after this generally made reference to cases occuring during pregnancy or in the post-partum period (Mannucci 2002).

1452–1519

During the pioneering atmosphere of the Rennaissance, dissection was accepted as a means to new discoveries (prior to this it was restricted, due to the belief that it was disrespectful to God). The anatomical drawings of Leonardo da Vinci (1452–1519) were some of the first to clearly document the structure of the venous system.

1628

Once dissection was established as a legitimate part of medical training, numerous new discoveries emerged. In 1628 William Harvey (1578–1657) overturned medical thinking by proving that blood circulates, and that the valves in veins are there to ensure unidirectional flow.

1644–1686

In 1644, Schenk first observed venous thrombosis when he described an occlusion in the inferior vena cava, and as early as 1686 the first theories on the aetiology of venous thrombosis were outlined by Richard Wiseman (1633–1714). He documented the case of a pharmacist's wife, who developed pain and swelling of her leg after a difficult labour and attributed the cause of the thrombosis to be systemic alteration in the circulating blood (pioneering the idea of 'hypercoagulability') – which he noted to be more prevalent in pregnancy and malignancy (Dickson 2004). The 'milk leg' of pregnancy was believed until the end of the eighteenth century to be due to the retention in the legs of unconsumed breast milk or commonly 'evil humours', and the French surgeon Ambroise Pare believed that leg swelling during pregnancy was due to the rention and concentration of menstrual blood (Mannucci 2002).

1800

Harvey's demonstration of blood cirulation led scientists Hunter, Baillie and Hewson to abandon the theory of retention of humours and adopt the concept that venous thrombosis was due to the closure of veins by blood clots. They proposed that slow blood flow was a likely cause of this and that the thrombus formed because of a 'coagulable lymph' in plasma (the substance that was later called fibrinogen; Hunter 1793; Baillie 1793; Hewson 1846). In 1800, Hull wrote the first literature review on venous thrombosis, for the first time calling it 'phlegmasia dolens', and surmised that the coagulation of 'lymph' was due to inflammation (Mannucci 2002).

1800–1860s

The risk factors for VTE were recognised at the turn of the nineteenth century. Ferrier (1810) noted that medical illness, particularly if associated with prolonged immobilization, was a risk factor and that the condition also occurred during debilitating infections such as typhus. Hodgson (1815) noted that injury to a vein might cause thrombosis and Hutchinson (1829) described a case of 'phlegmasia dolens' in a patient who had sustained a blow to the shin from a piece of timber (Anning 1957). Surgery was first recognized as a risk factor by Spencer Wells in 1866.

Towards the end of the nineteenth century, the pathologists Virchow and Rokitansky conducted autopsy studies on fatal cases of post-partum thrombosis and concluded, independently of one another, the famous three factors of 'Virchow's triad' [(vessel wall damage; decreased venous blood flow; and changes in blood leading to an increased tendency to clot formation (hypercoagulability)] as being the cause of venous thrombosis. In 1846, Virchow recognized the association between venous thrombosis in the legs and pulmonary embolism.

1860s–1900s

The components of Virchow's triad were well investigated over the next century, and with this research came new treatments. In Virchow's era, treatments had progressed from the blood letting of the Middle Ages to bed-rest and leeches. Surgical intervention to remove the thrombosed veins was advocated in the 1860s, then in 1884 it was discovered that leeches have anticoagulant properties (Dickson 2004). Following on from this, heparin was discovered as an anticoagulant in 1916, but was not introduced into clinical practice until the 1930s. Murray (1947) recognized its use in the prevention of PE in surgical patients. In the late 1940s the coumarins were introduced into the treatment of VTE, and De Takats (1950) suggested that the injection of a low-dose heparin would prevent DVT.

Our methods of detection improved in the 1930s, when venography was introduced to visualize the veins (Barber 1932) – a method that remains the 'gold standard' for detection but has been widely replaced today by the less invasive ultrasound.

1950 onwards

The 1950s were established as the era of thrombolysis, stemming from Astrup's finding of a substance in the tissues that was capable of activating the proteolytic enzymes in blood (Astrup 1951). This led to the discovery that streptokinase could dissolve intravascular thrombi (Johnson *et al.* 1952).

Our knowledge of genetic predisposition to clotting improved in the late twentieth century with the recognition of protein C and protein S deficiencies in the 1980s (Griffin *et al.* 1981; Comp *et al.* 1984). The 'factor V Leiden' mutation was discovered in the early 1990s (Bertina *et al.* 1994); this mutation leads to a hypercoagulable state and has since been found to be present in around 20% of patients who present with a first episode of VTE (Koster *et al.* 1993).

Conclusion

VTE is a significant problem in the United Kingdom today and our understanding of it continues to grow year by year as further research is completed. Although much has been discovered since Virchow, the value of a clinical diagnosis of VTE remains unchanged. History taking can identify risk factors but examination rarely gives us a definitive diagnosis. Today, detection of the problem is based on assessment of clinical risk and the judicious use of the investigations and treatment we now have available to us.

It is hoped that the chapters that follow will provide a comprehensive summary of VTE that can be read as a whole or as a reference point, enabling health professionals to consider VTE risk factors in their patients to provide them with up to date and effective care.

References

All Party Parliamentary Thrombosis Group (APPTG) (2007) *Thrombosis Awareness, Assessment, Management and Prevention. An Audit of Acute NHS Hospital Trusts.* November 2007. Available at: www.dvtreport.com

All Party Parliamentary Thrombosis Group (APPTG) (2008) *Thrombosis Awareness, Assessment, Management and Prevention. An Audit of Acute NHS Hospital Trusts.* November 2008. Available at: www.dvtreport.com

Anderson FA Jr, Wheeler HB, Goldberg RJ *et al.* (1991) A population-based perspective of the hospital incidence and case fatality rates of deep vein thrombosis and pulmonary embolism: the Worcester DVT Study. *Archives of Internal Medicine* **151**: 933–938.

Anderson FA Jr, Wheeler HB (1992) Physician practices in the management of venous thromboembolism, a community-wide survey. *Journal of Vascular Surgery* **16**: 707–714.

Anderson FA Jr (1995) Venous thromboembolism, risk factors and prophylaxis. *Clinics in Chest Medicine* **16**: 235–251.

Anderson FA Jr, Spencer FA (2003) Risk factors for venous thromboembolism. *Circulation* **107**: I-9-I-16.

Angchaisuksiri P, Pingsuthiwong S, Aryuchai K *et al.* (2000) Prevalence of the G1691A mutation in the factor V gene (factor V Leiden) and the *G20210A* prothrombin gene mutation in the Thai population. *American Journal of Hematology* **65**: 119–122.

Anning ST (1957) The historical aspects of venous thrombosis. *Medicine History* **1**: 28–37.

Astrup T (1951) The activation of a proteolytic enzyme in the blood by animal tissue. *Biochemistry Journal* **50**: 5.

Baillie J (1793) Of uncommon appearances of disease in blood vessels. *Transactions of the Society for the Improvement in Medical and Chirurgical Knowledge* **1**: 119.

Barber TH (1932) Some X-ray observations in varicose disease of the leg. *Lancet* **223**: 175–178.

Baron JA, Gridley G, Weiderpass E, Nyren O, Linet M (1998). *Venous thromboembolism and cancer Lancet* **351**: 1077–1080.

Bertina RM, Koeleman BP, Koster T *et al.* (1994) Mutation in blood coagulation factor V associated with resistance to activated protein C. *Nature* **369**: 64–67.

Bosanquet N (1992) Costs of venous ulcers, from maintenance therapy to investment programmes. *Phlebology* **1**(suppl 1): 44–46.

Boulay F, Berthier F, Schoukroun G *et al.* (2001) Seasonal variations in hospital admission for deep vein thrombosis and pulmonary embolism, analysis of discharge data. *British Medical Journal* **323**: 601–602.

Bounameaux H, Hicklin L, Desmarais S (1996) Seasonal variation in deep vein thrombosis. *British Medical Journal* **312**: 284–285.

Clagett GP, Anderson FA Jr, Geerts W *et al.*(1998) Prevention of venous thromboembolism. *Chest* **114**(5): 531–560S.

Chief Medical Officer (CMO) (2007) Sir Liam Donaldson's letter announcing the recommendations of the expert working group on the prevention of venous thromboembolism in hospitalised patients: http://www.dh.gov.uk/en/Publicationsandstatistics/Lettersandcirculars/Dearcolleagueletters/DH_073957

Comp PC, Esmon CT (1984) Recurrent venous thromboembolism in patients with a partial deficiency of protein S. *New England Journal of Medicine* **311**: 1525–1528.

Cushman M, Tsai AW, White RH *et al.* (2004) Deep vein thrombosis and pulmonary embolism in two cohorts: the longitudinal investigation of thromboembolism etiology. *American Journal of Medicine* **117**: 19–25.

Department of Health (DH) (2007) Report of the Independent Expert Working Group on the prevention of venous thromboembolism in hospitalised patients. DH, London. Available at: http://www.dh.gov.uk/en/Publicationsandstatistics/Publications/PublicationsPolicyAndGuidance/DH_073944

De Takats G (1950) Anticoagulation therapy in surgery. *Journal of the American Medical Association* **142**: 527.

Dexter L, Folch-Pi W (1974) Venous thrombosis, an account of the first documented case. *Journal of the American Medical Association* **228**: 195–196.

Dickson BC (2004) Venous thrombosis: on the history of Virchow's triad. *University of Toronto Medical Journal* **81**: 166–171.

Dismuke SE, Wagner EH (1986) Pulmonary embolism as a cause of death. The changing mortality in hospitalized patients. *Journal of the American Medical Association* **255**: 2039–2042.

Douketis JD, Kearon C, Bates S *et al.* (1998) Risk of fatal pulmonary embolism in patients with treated venous thromboembolism. *Journal of the American Medical Association* **279**: 458–462.

Ferrier J (1810) An affectation of the lymphatic vessels hitherto misunderstood. In *Medical Histories and Reflections*, Vol III.

Goldhaber SZ (1997) International cooperative pulmonary embolism registry detects high mortality rate. *Circulation* **96**(Suppl I), I-159.

Goldhaber SZ (1998) Pulmonary embolism. *New England Journal of Medicine* **339**: 93–104.

Goldhaber SZ, Visani L, De Rosa M (1999) Acute pulmonary embolism: clinical outcomes in the International Cooperative Pulmonary Embolism Registry (ICOPER). *Lancet* **353**: 1386–1389.

Goldhaber SZ (2004) Prevention of recurrent idiopathic venous thromboembolism. *Circulation* **110**: 20–24.

Gregg JP, Yamane AJ, Grody WW (1997) Prevalence of the factor V Leiden mutation in four distinct Am ethnic populations. *American Journal of Medical Genetics* **73**: 334–336.

Griffin JH, Evatt B, Zimmerman TS *et al.* (1981) Deficiency of protein C in congenital thrombotic disease. *Journal of Clinical Investigations* **68**: 1370–1373.

Heit JA, Silverstein MD, Mohr DN *et al.* (1999) Predictors of survival after deep vein thrombosis and pulmonary embolism. A population-based cohort study. *Archives of Internal Medicine* **159**(5): 445–453.

Heit J, Silverstein MD, Mohr DN *et al.* (2000) Predictors of recurrence after deep vein thrombosis and pulmonary embolism: a population based cohort study. *Archives of Internal Medicine* **160**: 761–768.

Heit JA, Melton LJ 3rd, Lohse CM *et al.* (2001) Incidence of venous thromboembolism in hospitalized patients versus community residents. *Mayo Clinic Proceedings* **76**: 1102–1110.

Heit JA (2005) Venous thromboembolism, disease burden, outcomes and risk factors. State of the art. *Journal of Thrombosis and Haemostasis* **3**: 1611–1617.

Heit J, Cohen AT, Anderson FA Jr (2005) Estimated annual number of incident and recurrent, non-fatal and fatal venous thromboembolism (VTE) events in the United States. *Blood* **106**: 267 (abstr).

Heit JA, Petterson T, Farmer S *et al.* (2006) Trends in incidence of deep vein thrombosis and pulmonary embolism: a 35-year population-based study. *Blood* **108**: 430a.

Heit JA (2008) Venous thromboembolism: mechanisms, treatment and public awareness. The epidemiology of venous thromboembolism in the community. *Arteriosclerosis, Thrombosis, and Vascular Biology* **28**: 370–372.

Hewson W (1846) *The Works of William Hewson FRS*, Gulliver Edition. Sydenham Society, London (cross-referenced from Mannucci, 2002)

Hodgson J (1815) *A Treatise on the diseases of arteries and veins*. Underwood. London.

Horlander KT, Mannino DM, Leeper KV (2003) Pulmonary embolism mortality in the United States 1979–1998: an analysis using multiple-cause mortality data. *Archives of Internal Medicine* **163**(14): 1711–1717.

House of Commons Health Committee (2005) *The Prevention of Venous Thromboembolism in Hospitalised Patients*. HC99. Stationery Office, London. Available at: www.publications.parliament.uk/pa/cm200405/cmselect/cmhealth/99/9902.htm*evidence_downloaded_29

Hunt BJ (2008) Awareness and politics of venous thromboembolism in the United Kingdom. *Arteriosclerosis, Thrombosis and Vascular Biology* **28**: 398–399.

Hunter J (1793) Observations on the inflammation of the internal coasts of veins. *Transactions of the Society for the Improvement of Medical and Chirurgical Knowledge* **1**: 18–25.

Hutchinson, AC (1829) In Lee, R. Pathological researches on inflammation of the veins of the uterus with additional observations on phlegmasia dolens. *Medico-Chirurgical Transactions* **XV**: 425.

Johnson AJ, Tillett WS (1952) The lysis in rabbits of intravascular blood clots by streptococcal fibrinolytic system (streptokinase). *Journal of Experimental Medicine* **95**: 449–464.

Kearon C (2003) Natural history of venous thromboembolism. *Circulation* **107**: I-22–I-30.

Klatsky AL, Armstrong MA, Poggi J (2000) Risk of pulmonary embolism and/or deep vein thrombosis in Asian-Americans. *American Journal of Cardiology* **85**: 1334–1337.

Koster T, Rosendaal FR, de Ronde H *et al.* (1993) Venous thrombosis due to poor anticoagulant response to activated protein C: Leiden Thrombophilia Study. *Lancet* **342**: 1503–1506.

Laporte S, Mismetti P, Décousus H *et al.* (2008) Clinical predictors for fatal pulmonary embolism in 15520 patients with venous thromboembolism. *Circulation* **117**: 1711–1716.

Laing W (1992) *Chronic Venous Diseases of the Leg.* Office of Health Economics, London.

Lindblad B, Erikson A, Bergquist D (1991) Incidence of venous thromboembolism verified by necropsy over 30 years. *British Medical Journal* **302**, 709–711.

Mannucci PM (2002) Venous thrombosis: the history of knowledge. *Pathophysiology Haemostasis and Thrombosis* **32**: 209–212.

McRae S, Tran H, Schulman S *et al.* (2006) Effect of patient's sex on risk of recurrent venous thromboembolism: a meta-analysis. *Lancet* **368**: 371–378.

Murray G (1947) Anticoagulants in venous thrombosis and the prevention of pulmonary embolism. *Surgery, Gynecology and Obstetrics* **106**: 898–906.

Nordstrom M, Lindblad B, Bergqvist D *et al.* (1992) A prospective study of the incidence of deep-vein thrombosis within a defined urban population. *Journal of Internal Medicine* **232**: 155–160.

Oger E (2000) Incidence of venous thromboembolism, a community-based study in Western France. EPI–GETBP Study Group. Groupe d'Etude de la Thrombose de Bretagne Occidentale. *Thrombosis and Haemostasis* **83**: 657–660.

Palareti G, Cosmi B, Legnani C *et al.* (2006) D-dimer testing to determine the duration of anticoagulation therapy. *New England Journal of Medicine* **355**: 1780–1789.

Pearce JMS (2002) Rudolf Ludwig Karl Virchow (1821–1902). *Journal of Neurology* **249**: 492–493.

Prandoni P, Lensing AWA, Prins MH *et al.* (2002) Residual venous thrombosis as a predictive factor of recurrent venous thromboembolism. *Annals of Internal Medicine* **137**: 955–960.

Ridker PM, Miletich JP, Hennekens CH *et al.* (1997) Ethnic distribution of factor V Leiden in 4047 men and women. Implications for venous thromboembolism screening. *Journal of the American Medical Association* **277**: 1305–1307.

Safavi-Abbasi S, Reis C, Talley MC *et al.* (2006) Rudolf Ludwig Karl Virchow: pathologist, physician, anthropologist, and politician. *Neurosurgical Focus* **20**: 1–6.

Sandler DA, Martin JF (1989) Autopsy proven pulmonary embolism in hospital patients: are we detecting enough deep vein thrombosis? *Journal of the Royal Society of Medicine* **82**: 203–205.

Schulman S, Lindmarker P, Holmström M *et al.* (2006) Post-thrombotic syndrome: recurrence and death 10 years after the first episode of venous thromboembolism treated with warfarin for 6 weeks or 6 months. *Journal of Thrombosis and Haemostasis* **4**: 732–742.

Siddique RM, Siddique MI, Connors AF Jr *et al.* (1996) Thirty-day case-fatality rates for pulmonary embolism in the elderly. *Archives of Internal Medicine* **156**: 2343–2347.

Silverstein MD, Heit JA, Mohr DN *et al.* (1998) Trends in the incidence of deep vein thrombosis and pulmonary embolism: a 25-year population-based study. *Archives of Internal Medicine* **158**: 585–593.

Verstraete M (1997) Prophylaxis of venous thromboembolism. *British Medical Journal* **314**: 123–125.

Virchow RLK (1847) Ueber die akute Entzuendung der Arterien. *Archiv fur pathologische Anatomie und Physiologie und fur klinische Medizin Berlin* **1**: 272–274.

Virchow RLK (1978) *Cellular Pathology*, 1859 Special Edition. John Churchill, London: 204–207.

White RH, Zhou H, Romano PS (1998) Incidence of idiopathic deep venous thrombosis and secondary thromboembolism among ethnic groups in California. *Annals of Internal Medicine* **128**: 737–740.

White RH (2003) The epidemiology of venous thromboembolism. *Circulation* **107**(Suppl 1): I4–8.

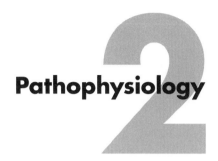

Pathophysiology

Overview

To fully understand VTE, it is necessary to return to the basic sciences of anatomy, physiology and pathophysiology. Chapter 2 covers the anatomy of the venous system specific to the lower limbs and touches on the physiology of blood flow. The constituents of Virchow's triad are broken down and discussed in detail to provide an understanding of the pathophysiology of VTE. Normal coagulation and 'the coagulation cascade' is introduced and explained, with clinical correlation to risk factors for VTE.

Anatomy of the lower limb veins

The veins of the leg are divided into a superficial and deep vein group (Figure 2.1). The greater and lesser saphenous veins are subcutaneous and form the superficial system. They are separated from the deep system by the fascia. Connecting veins run through the fascia to connect the two systems. Normally 80% of the venous drainage of the leg is transported in the deep veins and 20% in the superficial veins (Diehm

Venous Thromboembolism: A Nurses Guide to Prevention and Management   By Ellen Welch
© 2010 John Wiley & Sons, Ltd.

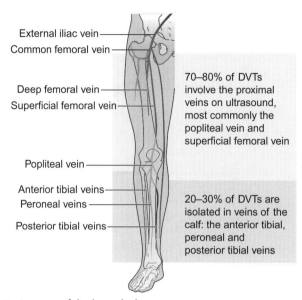

External iliac vein

Common femoral vein

Deep femoral vein

Superficial femoral vein

70–80% of DVTs involve the proximal veins on ultrasound, most commonly the popliteal vein and superficial femoral vein

Popliteal vein

Anterior tibial veins

Peroneal veins

Posterior tibial veins

20–30% of DVTs are isolated in veins of the calf: the anterior tibial, peroneal and posterior tibial veins

Figure 2.1 Anatomy of the lower limb veins.

et al. 2000). The deep veins accompany the arteries and usually take on the name of the artery they run with – they can also be known as venae commitantes, which is Latin for 'accompanying vein'.

The deep veins of the calf consist of three pairs of veins: the anterior tibial veins, the posterior tibial veins and the peroneal veins. Each of these veins divides into several trunks surrounding the artery and these anastomose freely with each other. The anterior tibial veins drain blood from the dorsum of the foot, while the posterior tibial veins are formed by the meeting of the superficial and deep plantar veins. The peroneal veins are found behind the fibula. Together, these veins are known as the stem veins of the calf. The stem veins all unite to form the popliteal vein. There are two types of veins in the calf muscles: 'sinusoidal veins', which are large, valveless veins joining the posterior tibial and peroneal veins (commonly found in the soleal muscle); and thin and straight veins with valves, predominating in the gastrocnemius muscles. The calf muscle veins drain into the popliteal vein. It has been demonstrated using phlebography that calf vein thrombosis is as likely to originate in stem veins as from the soleal muscle veins (Thomas *et al.* 1977).

In the thigh, the popliteal vein changes its name to become the femoral vein. It joins with the deep femoral vein at the proximal thigh to become the common femoral vein, running parallel with the femoral

Box 2.1 May–Thurner syndrome

DVT is thought to occur three to eight times more often in the left leg than in the right (Cockett *et al.* 1965; Patel *et al.* 2000), Dissections carried out on 412 cadavers in the 1940s discovered obstructive lesions in 23.8% of left common iliac veins, which were composed of elastin and collagen rather than clot (Ehrich *et al.* 1943). In 1957 May and Thurner reported an iliac compression syndrome, describing an impedance to venous flow resulting from intimal changes in the vessel (May *et al.* 1957). It was found that proliferation of the endothelium of the vessel was caused by compression of the left common iliac vein by the right common iliac artery, which caused the walls of the vein to rub against each other. An early diagnosis of iliac vein compression can prevent progression to thrombosis and venous insufficiency syndrome and the condition should be suspected in patients with a history of persistent left leg swelling, with or without DVT, with no obvious cause (Barbarose 2004). Venography confirms the diagnosis and the mechanical compression should be relieved by either direct surgical repair or endovascular stent placement to prevent DVT (Patel *et al.* 2000). It is thought that many cases of left iliofemoral thrombosis associated with May–Thurner syndrome are missed due to the replacement of venography with ultrasound, therefore the true prevalence of the disorder is unknown (Taheri *et al.* 1987).

arteries up to the inguinal ligament, where the common femoral vein becomes the external iliac vein. The blood from the legs drains into the inferior vena cava via the external and common iliac veins. The external and internal iliac veins join at the level of the sacroiliac joint to become the common iliac vein. The junction of the left common iliac vein with the inferior vena cava is longer and more oblique than the right and has been found a common site for the development of leg and pelvic thrombosis (see Box 2.1).

Veins

Like arteries, the deep veins contain three layers, of muscle fibres, elastin and collagen, the outer tunica adventitia, the middle tunica media and the inner tunica intima. Because of the lower blood pressure in the venous system, the walls of veins are much thinner than those of arteries, with less muscle and elastic tissue (Box 2.2). Veins in the extremities, which have to work against gravity to return the blood to

---

Box 2.2 Differences between veins and arteries

Vein

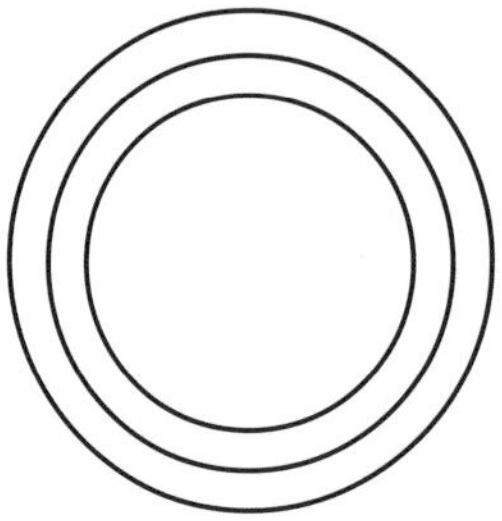

Artery

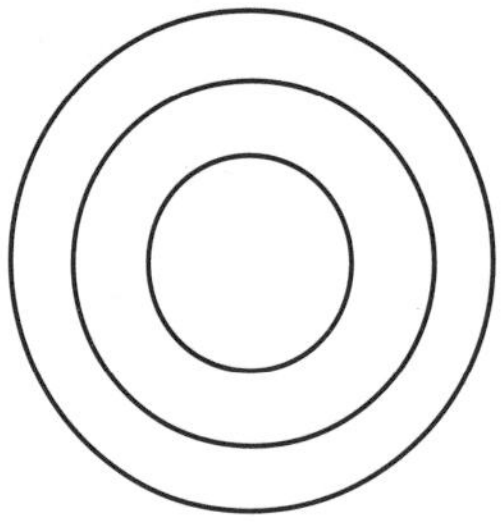

Veins

- Have wide lumens (see diagram above) with relatively less muscle and elastic tissue.
- Have valves to prevent back flow of blood.
- Transport deoxygenated blood back towards the heart under lower pressure than arteries.

Arteries

- Have narrow lumens (see diagram above) and relatively more muscle and elastic tissue.
- Do not have valves (except for the semi-lunar valves of the pulmonary artery and the aorta).
- Transport oxygenated blood away from the heart under higher pressure.

---

the heart, are fitted with valves, which direct blood flow back to the heart. Valves are made up of a strong layer of collagen fibres covered with endothelium and occur approximately every 2 cm in the deep veins of the calves. The sinusoidal veins of the soleal muscle have no valves (Browse *et al.* 1988).

The calf muscle pump, alternatively known as 'the peripheral heart', aids this delivery of blood back to the heart. When the calf muscles contract, the deep veins of the leg are compressed, which forces the blood back to the central circulation. Reflux of blood is prevented by the venous valves. During muscle relaxation, the superficial leg veins drain into the deep veins. Pump failure is caused by weakness of the muscles, incompetent valves and obstruction of the vessels by extensive thrombosis, which leads to chronic venous insufficiency and venous hypertension. The arm muscles produce a similar pumping effect but, as the hydrostatic pressure in the arms is lower, venous malfunction never causes the skin changes and ulceration which occur with similar malfunction in the lower limbs (Browse *et al.* 1988).

Virchow's triad

The three factors that contribute towards venous thrombosis will be discussed in turn, with relevance to the underlying pathophysiology:

1. Venous stasis
2. Venous trauma
3. Hypercoagulability

The risk factors, which are described in Chapter 3, all fall into one or more of the categories above, often with some overlap. The more risk factors a person has, the greater his/her risk of a thrombus developing.

Venous stasis

Most venous thrombi seem to originate in areas of slow blood flow, such as the large venous sinuses of the calf and thigh, or in valve cusp pockets (Nicolaides *et al.* 1971). There are also a number of conditions which cause defective venous drainage and are known to be associated with an increased risk of VTE – supporting the theory that stasis is a causative factor. These conditions include left common iliac vein compression syndrome (see Box 2.1), paralysed calf muscles (Myllynen *et al.* 1985), partial vena cava obstruction during pregnancy (Kerr *et al.* 1964) and iliac vein obstruction following kidney transplant (Joffe 1976).

When patients are immobile, especially during surgery and the postoperative period, there is a reduction in muscle contraction, which reduces the efficiency of the 'calf muscle pump' and therefore the amount of blood returned from the legs. Stagnant blood then can trigger endothelial wall damage and subsequent thrombus formation.

Postoperative immobile patients are at an increased risk of VTE, especially if they remain immobile after discontinuation of thromboprophylaxis (Sigel *et al.* 1974; Gallus *et al.* 1976). Autopsy studies have shown a greater incidence of VTE in those patients confined to bedrest for more than a week and in those patients with fractures of the lower limbs immobilized in plaster cast – all factors promoting venous stasis (Gibbs 1957; Hamilton *et al.* 1970).

Blood flow is also thought to be hindered by increased blood viscosity. Blood becomes thicker in a number of disease conditions, such as polycythaemia and the dysproteinaemias, and during periods of dehydration (Mammen 1992). Certain inflammatory diseases can result in patients having increased fibrinogen levels (fibrinogen is a sticky acute phase reactant protein, which promotes thrombosis by causing platelets to clump together in vessels) and it has been found that fibrinogen levels are also increased in patients with spinal cord injury and paralysis (Rossi *et al.* 1980). Higher levels of fibrinogen may also contribute to venous stasis, resulting in an increased risk of VTE.

Venous trauma

It was discovered as early as 1922 that there was an increase in blood fibrinogen in response to trauma (Foster *et al.* 1922). Since then it has been found that the endothelium of the vessel wall plays an important role in clotting (see below). The endothelium produces a huge array of substances (prostacyclin, bradykinin, angiotensin, adenonucleotides, plasminogen activator, tissue urokinase, factor VIII-related protein, glycosaminoglycans) that are thought to prevent the deposition of thrombi or have local effects on coagulation and fibrinolysis (Mason *et al.* 1977). 'Heparin-like' glycosaminoglycans receptors have been identified on the surface of the endothelium that seem to play an important anticoagulant role in non-damaged vessel walls, which, when disturbed by trauma, appear to activate the clotting system (Mammen 1992). Defective production or release of tissue plasminogen activator appear to be associated with recurrent DVT (Stead *et al.* 1983). Further research is needed to determine the exact roles of the different substances and the parts they play in thrombus formation.

Endothelial damage to the vein wall can also occur due to venous stasis. Stasis can cause back-flow of blood and dilatation of the venous valves, which can lead to tearing of the endothelium layer. The damaged wall releases factors which can activate the clotting cascade, leading to increased thrombosis (Coleridge-Smith 1990).

It is known that microscopic vessel wall damage occurs in patients undergoing hip or knee replacement surgery (Stamatakis *et al.* 1977) and, in the absence of thromboprophylaxis, hip fracture surgery carries a high risk of VTE (Gillespie *et al.* 2000).

Hypercoagulability

The coagulation system is made up of a clotting and a fibrinolytic system (see below). An imbalance in either system will result in either a tendency to bleed or a tendency to clot. Patients prone to thrombosis will have either an inhibited fibronolytic system or a hyperactive clotting system.

A decrease in the substances that usually break down clots, such as protein C, protein S and antithrombin, will result in an increased t endency to clot – such deficiencies are usually inherited. In over 50% of patients presenting with juvenile or idiopathic VTE, an inherited thrombophilic condition can be identified (Anderson *et al.* 2003). Anti-thrombin deficiency was first identified in the 1960s (Egeberg 1965), then in the 1980s protein C and protein S deficiencies were recognized (Griffin *et al.* 1981; Comp *et al.* 1984). The discovery of activated protein C resistance by Dahlback *et al.* (1993) led to the discovery of a mutation in the factor V gene, know as factor V Leiden, which has since been found to be the most prevalent hereditary thrombophilia (Koster *et al.* 1993). Elevated levels of several coagulation factors, including factors VIII, IX and XI, have been linked with an increased thrombotic risk, although the mechanism of action is unclear (Anderson *et al.* 2003). Another commonly encountered acquired abnormality associated with increased VTE is the presence of anticardiolipin antibodies and lupus anticoagulants, known as antiphospholipid antibody syndrome. Ginsberg *et al.* (1992) showed that patients with anticardiolipin antibody titres above the 95th percentile had a 5.3-fold increased risk of developing DVT or PE over a five year period.

Patients with congenital thrombophilia generally remain asymptomatic until their clotting system faces a major challenge, such as surgery or childbirth, again suggesting that it is a combination of the factors of Virchow's triad that leads to VTE formation (Mammen 1992). The inherited thrombophilias and antiphospholipid syndrome are explained in Box 2.3.

Venous thrombus formation

Venous thrombosis is a condition in which a blood clot (thrombus) forms inappropriately in a vein. This manifests clinically as deep vein thrombosis (DVT), commonly in the deep veins of the legs, thighs and

Box 2.3 Blood disorders causing hypercoagulability

Factor V Leiden (activated protein C resistance)

Activated protein C (aPC) in conjunction with protein S are natural inhibitors of coagulation – they inactivate both factor Va and factor VIIIa. Factor V is a proenzyme that is activated to factor Va to cata-lyse the activation of prothrombin to thrombin, which leads to clot formation. In 1993 in Holland, Dahlback *et al.*, through a series of experiments, discovered aPC resistance, which was eventually found to be due to a mutation in the gene for factor V, named factor V Leiden after the city in The Netherlands where it was first identi-fied (Bertina *et al.* 1994). Factor V Leiden is the most prevalent hereditary thrombophilia among white Europeans (De Stefano *et al.* 1998) and 20–60% of patients with recurrent VTE display APC resistance on laboratory testing (Koster *et al.* 1993). Patients with the factor V Leiden mutation have a factor V variant which cannot be degraded as easily by aPC. Factor V therefore remains active, which leads to overproduction of thrombin, leading to excess clot-ting. Prolonged or lifelong therapy with oral anticoagulants is con-sidered even after a single thrombotic event (Zoller *et al.* 1999).

Protein C deficiency

Clot formation depends on thrombin generation and in the normal clotting cascade, protein C inhibits thrombin generation. Deficiency of protein C therefore results in venous thrombosis. In the rare inherited homozygous (two copies of the defective gene inherited one from each parent) state, this deficiency is associated with massive venous thrombosis or life-threatening neonatal purpura fulminans. The inherited heterozygous (one copy of the defective gene inherited) state is present in 2–5% of thrombosis patients (Zoller *et al.* 1999) and is associated with lower limb DVT, but a significant number of patients remain asymptomatic. Patients are generally given anticoagulant therapy in situations that put them at an increased risk for VTE. Prolonged or lifelong therapy with oral anticoagulants is considered after even a single thrombotic event . Acquired states of protein C deficiency occur during severe sepsis and DIC and may require treatment with protein C concentrates.

Protein S deficiency

Protein S is a vitamin K-dependent anticoagulant protein which functions as a cofactor to facilitate the action of activated protein

C. Deficiency of protein S is an autosomal dominant disease present in 2–5% of patients with thrombosis (Zoller *et al.* 1999). The homozygous state occurs rarely and those patients present early in life with purpura fulminans. Acquired deficiencies of protein S can occur with liver disease, vitamin K deficiency or as a result of commencing therapy with oral vitamin K antagonists. Sickle cell anaemia and pregnancy can both cause decreased levels of protein S (Francis 1988). Patients with protein S deficiency who develop thrombosis should be initially anticoagulated with heparin for a minimum of five days, followed by oral warfarin therapy.

Antithrombin III deficiency

Antithrombin III inhibits the coagulation cascade by lysing thrombin and factor Xa. Heparin exerts its anticoagulant effect by potentiating the action of antithrombin III. Congenital antithrombin III deficiency occurs when an individual inherits either one or two defective genes. Acquired antithrombin III deficiency is due to consumption of antithrombin and occurs when the coagulation system is inappropriately activated, such as during disseminated intravascular coagulation (DIC). Loss of antithrombin III can occur during periods of increased protein catabolism or secondary to nephrotic syndrome. Treatment depends on the presentation. Patients with a congenital deficiency who develop thrombosis require indefinite anticoagulation with warfarin therapy. Heparin activity is not as reliable in patients with antithrombin III deficiency, so careful monitoring of the anti-Xa activity is required. In acquired antithrombin III deficiency, the underlying cause should be established and corrected. Replacement using antithrombin III concentrates is the usual approach.

Prothrombin G20210A

Prothrombin (also known as factor II) is a vitamin K-dependent coenzyme that is cleaved by factor Xa to form thrombin. The prothrombin 20210a gene mutation results in increased levels of plasma prothrombin and an associated two- to threefold increased risk of thrombosis (Poort *et al.* 1996). The mutation can be identified without DNA analysis and should be done as part of a thrombophilia screen. Oral contraceptives should be avoided in women who carry the mutation. Carriers have an increased risk of recurrent DVT after a first episode and are therefore candidates for lifelong treatment with oral anticoagulants (De Stefano *et al.* 1999).

Antiphospholipid syndrome

This is an autoimmune disorder of unknown cause, characterized by recurrent arterial and venous thrombosis and/or recurrent fetal losses, combined with high levels of circulating anticardiolipin antibodies and the presence of the lupus anticoagulant (Levine *et al.* 2002). Patients known to have antiphospholipid syndrome should eliminate other VTE risk factors, such as oral contraceptives and smoking. Once thrombosis is established, treatment is as normal with heparin and warfarin therapy, with a target INR of 2.0–3.0 for venous thrombosis and 3.0 for arterial thrombosis. Patients with recurrent thrombi despite anticoagulation should aim for a higher INR of 3.0–4.0 (Lim *et al.* 2006).

Hyperhomocysteinemia

This is a blood disorder caused by elevated levels of the amino acid homocysteine in the blood, which is linked to an increased risk of cardiovascular disease and also VTE. In the Leiden thrombophilia study, 10% of the 269 patients with DVT had significantly elevated homocysteine levels (Den Heijer *et al.* 1996). It is thought that homocysteine may have a toxic effect on the vascular endothelium and on the clotting cascade but the exact causative mechanisms are unclear (Rees *et al.* 1993). Folic acid and vitamins B6 and B12 can lower homocysteine levels, but further research is required to determine whether this therapy will contribute to the prevention of VTE (Den Heijer *et al.* 1994).

pelvis. If fragments of thrombi (known as emboli) break off, they can lodge in vessels downstream. A blood clot that comes to rest in the vessels of the pulmonary arterial system and blocks the flow of blood through the lungs is known as a pulmonary embolism (PE) and a large PE can be fatal (Blann *et al.* 2006). DVT and PE are collectively known as venous thromboembolism (VTE).

The lungs provide such an effective filter that the venous and arterial systems are separate from the point of view of thromboembolism (except in patients with patent foramen ovale or atrial septal defect). Blood flow is faster in arteries than in veins, so although arterial thrombosis does occur, it is less common than venous thrombosis. It usually occurs in association with atheroma, which generally occurs in areas of turbulent blood flow. Arterial thrombi are commonly formed in the heart following myocardial infarction, on the surfaces of prosthetic valves and in the left atrium in mitral valve disease. Dislodged arterial thrombi can manifest clinically as an acutely ischaemic limb or a stroke.

Thrombus formation is a result of an imbalance between the antico-agulant and procoagulant systems in the blood (Enders *et al.* 2002). Three pathological processes, known collectively as Virchow's triad, have been shown to promote this imbalance, as outlined above (Virchow 1852). Patients with venous trauma (problems with the endothelial vessel wall), venous stasis (problems with blood flow) or hypercoagu-lability (problems with the blood's clotting components, which alter blood consistency) are predisposed to formation of VTE. Risk factors for VTE (covered in Chapter 3) alter one or more components of Vir-chow's triad. To understand how thrombus formation comes about, it is helpful to understand normal clotting mechanisms.

Haemostasis

Haemostasis or clot formation is a complex process that prevents death from blood loss when blood vessels are damaged. It depends upon interaction between platelets, clotting factors and the vessel wall. Under normal circumstances, the coagulation system is balanced in favour of anticoagulation (Dahlback 2000). If this tightly controlled series of events occurs in the wrong place at the wrong time, it can manifest as thrombosis. It may be helpful to break haemostasis into two phases: the initial primary phase, involving vascular constriction and platelet plug formation in response to the vessel damage; and fol-lowing this the secondary formation of a supportive fibrin mesh gener-ated by the coagulation pathway (Furie *et al.* 2005).

Primary haemostasis

Trauma to the vessel wall endothelial cells exposes the collagen found in the underlying subendothelium. Platelets become activated by this to extend pseudopodia, which allow them to adhere to the suben-dothelium and also to other platelets. This platelet binding depends on the presence of collagen in the vessel wall, glycoprotein membrane receptors on the surface of the platelets and a plasma protein secreted from endothelial cells, called von Willebrand factor (vWF), which mediates the adhesion of the platelets to the subendothelium (George 2000).

Following adhesion to the wall, platelets change shape to become spherical and release the contents of their cytoplasm, which include vWF, fibrinogen and other factors. The presence of the cytoplasmic contents encourages platelets to aggregate together. Plasma protein fibrinogen binds to the glycoprotein membrane receptors of platelets, cross-linking them together. The resulting mass of aggregated platelets plugs the breach in the vessel wall and provides an expanse of platelet membrane on which further coagulation reactions can continue.

Secondary haemostasis

The primary phase described above occurs within minutes of vessel damage, and the platelet plug formed will disintegrate unless it becomes strengthened by an insoluble fibrin net produced by the complex coagulation cascade during secondary haemostasis.

The coagulation cascade consists of a series of enzymatic reactions that ultimately result in the conversion of soluble plasma fibrinogen into a fibrin clot. The coagulation factors are predominantly produced in the liver and are identified by roman numerals (except for I, called fibrinogen; and II, called prothrombin. III, IV and VI are redundant). Factor V is also produced in platelets and endothelial cells. The coagulation factors circulate in their inactive form and, when activated, each is capable of further activating more components of the cascade. Active forms are denoted by 'a'. Factors XII, XI, X, IX and thrombin are enzyme precursors and factors V and VIII are cofactors (Kumar 2005).

The coagulation pathway (Figure 2.2)

Traditionally, this series of enzymatic reactions is divided into 'extrinsic' and 'intrinsic' pathways – a concept that remains useful when interpreting laboratory clotting tests (Box 2.4) but can be misleading, since in reality the two pathways are linked.

Coagulation is initiated by tissue factor (TF), a glycoprotein exposed on damaged vessels. TF binds to and activates factor VII, which in turn binds to and activates factor X. This part of the reaction was traditionally termed the 'extrinisic' pathway. Activated factor X stimulates the conversion of prothrombin to thrombin, which hydrolyses the peptide bonds of fibrinogen to form fibrin.

Unfortunately, the reaction between TF and VIIa is insufficient by itself to fully activate factor X, but it does activate factor IX, which then activates factor VIII to initiate the crucial activation of factor X. The reactions that follow are known as 'the common pathway'. Activated factor X forms a complex with factor V on the surface of the activated platelets, which allows the conversion of prothrombin to thrombin. Thrombin then converts fibrinogen into fibrin. At the same time, factor XIII is activated by thrombin in the presence of calcium ions to cross-link adjacent fibrin molecules, which stabilizes the clot (Weitz *et al.* 2004).

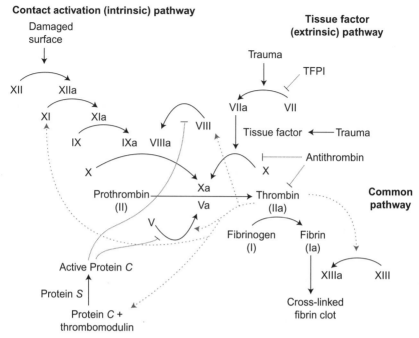

Figure 2.2 The coagulation cascade.

Box 2.4 Testing coagulation clinically

Prothrombin time (PT) tests the tissue factor (TF)-driven 'extrinsic' pathway and is prolonged with deficiencies of VII, X, V, II and fibrinogen and also if the patient is on warfarin or has liver disease. PT is usually expressed as a ratio, the international normalized ratio (INR), to account for different 'normal values' in different laboratories so as to aid the interpretation of results.

Activated partial thromboplastin time (APTT) tests the 'intrinsic' pathway and is prolonged with deficiencies of factors XII, XI, IX, VIII, X, V, II or fibrinogen.

Haemophilia results from a deficiency of factor VIII (A) or IX (B), the factors mainly responsible for the generation of thrombin. Both types are inherited as an X-linked disorder and clinical features ranging from mild bleeding after injury to spontaneous cerebral haemorrhage are dependent on the level of deficiency. Patients typically have a prolonged APTT and normal PT, bleeding time and vWF level. Treatment involves administration of the deficient factor.

A number of mechanisms are in place to prevent inappropriate activation of the coagulation pathway, and abnormalities of these can lead to an increased tendency towards thrombosis. Natural inhibitors of the activated coagulation factors circulate in the blood, the major players being antithrombin (AT) and activated protein C (aPC). AT is produced by the liver and has weak inhibitory action against thrombin and factor Xa. When AT binds with heparin, this activity is markedly increased (Dahlback 2000). aPC is generated from its vitamin K-dependent precursor, protein C. If thrombin forms around healthy vascular endothelial cells, inhibitory mechanisms are initiated and thrombin binds to the cell receptor thrombomodulin. This reaction enhances the activation of protein C, which ultimately inhibits factors Va and VIIIa, which reduces further thrombin generation. aPC relies on the presence of a cofactor, protein S. This information becomes clinically relevant when using anticoagulant medications such as warfarin (Box 2.5).

A clots also contains the seed of its own destruction, an inactive plasma protein called plasminogen. In a process known as fibrinolysis, plasminogen is converted by tissue plasminogen activator (tPA) secreted by healthy vascular endothelial cells into the fibrinolytic enzyme plasmin. Plasmin breaks down fibrinogen and fibrin into fibrin degradation products (FDPs; which include the D-dimer fragment, from the breakdown of cross-linked fibrin) and activates repair of the original vessel damage.

When clotting goes wrong – disseminated intravascular coagulation (DIC)

Also known as 'consumptive coagulopathy', this serious disorder is characterized by intravascular coagulation and bleeding. It is always triggered by an underlying disorder, such as sepsis, trauma and malignancy (the list of associated disorders is extensive). The coagulation system becomes activated, so that clotting is no longer localized to the area of need and, instead, widespread activation of the coagulation system occurs, resulting in the breakdown of fibrin and the consumption of coagulation factors. Thrombin generation results in the formation of small fibrin clots, which are deposited in the microcirculation and can cause end-organ damage. Activation of the fibrinolytic system can result in uncontrolled bleeding. The clinical features vary, depending on the underlying cause, but both bleeding and thrombosis can occur simultaneously. Typical laboratory results will show a prolonged PT with a low platelet count and a low fibrinogen level. D-dimer levels are usually elevated (Taylor *et al.* 2001). Treatment relies on sup-

Box 2.5 Vitamin K and warfarin (refer to Chapter 7 for further information)

Vitamin K is an essential cofactor required for the proper functioning of the coagulation pathway; without it coagulation factors cannot become 'activated'. Factors II, VII, IX and X and also protein S and protein C contain glutamic acid residues that must be carboxylated to generate an active catalytic site. Vitamin K acts as a cofactor in this reaction. The coumarin drug warfarin displays its anticoagulant properties by interfering with vitamin K metabolism.

The carboxylation reaction will only proceed if the carboxylase enzyme is able to convert a reduced form of vitamin K to vitamin K epoxide at the same time. The vitamin K epoxide is in turn recycled back to vitamin K by the enzyme vitamin K epoxide reductase. Warfarin inhibits this enzyme (Whitlon *et al.* 1978), reducing the available vitamin K in the tissues. The clotting factors are still produced but are biologically inactive, therefore blood clotting is diminished. Ironically, when warfarin is first initiated in patients it promotes clot formation, which is why heparin is often co-administered when starting warfarin. This is due to protein S, which is also dependent on vitamin K activity. Reduced levels of protein S lead to a reduction in protein C activity and therefore reduced inhibition of factor Va and factor VIIIa. This causes the coagulation pathway to be temporarily biased towards thrombus formation. Deficiency of vitamin K due to malabsorption or liver disease can also disrupt blood clotting (Kumar *et al.* 2005).

portive measures and management of the underlying illness. Each case should be considered individually, but treatment consists of the replacement of blood components and anticoagulants and antifibronolytics may be required (Levi *et al.* 1999).

Conclusion

After reading this chapter, you should feel confident to discuss the elements of Virchow's triad and understand how an imbalance in one or more of the three factors can lead to thrombus formation. The anatomy of the lower limbs and of the veins should be familiar and you should have some knowledge of the coagulation cascade,

Knowledge of these underlying mechanisms will enable a greater understanding of why DVT and PE occurs in certain patient groups and why certain treatment and prevention measures are used.

References

Anderson FA, Spencer FA (2003) Risk factors for venous thromboembolism. *Circulation* **107**: 9–16.

Barbarose EC (2004) Diagnosis please. Case 76: May–Thurner syndrome. *Radiology* **233**: 361–365.

Bertina RM, Koeleman BP, Koster T *et al.* (1994) Mutation in blood coagulation factor V associated with resistance to activated protein C. *Nature* **369**: 64–67.

Blann AD, Lip GY (2006) Venous thromboembolism. *British Medical Journal* **332**: 215–219.

Browse NL, Burnand KG, Thomas ML (1988) Physiology and functional anatomy. In *Diseases of the Veins: Pathology, Diagnosis and Treatment*, 1st Edition. Arnold, London.

Cockett FB, Thomas ML (1965) The iliac compression syndrome. *British Journal of Surgery* **52**: 816–821.

Coleridge-Smith PD (1990) Venous stasis and vein lumen changes during surgery. *British Journal of Surgery* **77**: 1055–1059.

Comp P, Esmon C (1984) Recurrent venous thromboembolism in patients with a partial deficiency of protein S. *New England Journal of Medicine* **311**: 1525–1528.

Dahlback B, Carlsson M, Svensson PJ (1993) Familial thrombophilia due to a previously unrecognised mechanism characterised by poor anticoagulant response to activated protein C: prediction of a cofactor to activated protein C. *Proceedings of the National Academy of Science of the United States of America* **90**: 1004–1008.

Dahlback B (2000) Blood coagulation. *Lancet* **355**: 1627–1632.

Den Heijer M, Bos GMJ, Gerrits WBJ *et al.* (1994) Will a decrease of blood homocysteine by vitamin supplementation reduce the risk for vascular disease? *Fibrinolysis* **8**: 91–92.

Den Heijer M, Koster T, Blom HJ *et al.* (1996) Hyperhomocysteinemia as a risk factor for deep vein thrombosis. *New England Journal of Medicine* **334**: 759–762.

De Stefano V, Chiusolo P, Paciaroni K *et al.* (1998) Epidemiology of factor V Leiden: clinical implications. *Seminars in Thrombosis and Hemostasis* **24**: 367–379.

De Stefano V, Martinelli I, Mannuccio P *et al.* (1999) The risk of recurrent deep venous thrombosis among heterozygous carriers of both factor V Leiden and the *G20210A* prothrombin mutation. *New England Journal of Medicine* **341**: 801–806.

Diehm C, Allenberg JR, Nimura-Eckert K *et al.* (2000) Diseases of veins. In *Color Atlas of Vascular Diseases*, 1st Edition. Springer-Verlag, Milan.

Egeberg O (1965) Inherited antithrombin deficiency causing thrombophilia. *Thrombosis et Diathesis Haemorrhagica* **13**: 516.

Enders JM, Burke, JM, Dobesh, PP (2002) Prevention of venous thromboembolism in acute medical illness. *Pharmacotherapy* **22**: 1564–1578.

Ehrich WE, Krumbhaar EB (1943) A frequent obstructive anomaly of the mouth of the left common iliac vein. *American Heart Journal* **26**: 737–750.

Foster DP, Whipple CH (1922) Blood fibrin studies. Fibrin influenced by cell injury, inflammation, intoxication, liver injury and the Eck fistula. Notes connecting the origin of fibrin in the body. *American Journal of Physiology* **58**: 407.

Francis RB (1988) Protein S deficiency in sickle cell anemia. *Journal of Laboratory Clinical Medicine* **111**: 571–576.

Furie B, Furie BC (2005) Thrombus formation *in vivo*. *Journal of Clinical Investigation* **115**: 3355–3362.

Gallus AS, Hirsh J, O'Brien SE *et al.* (1976) Prevention of deep vein thrombosis with small subcutaneous doses of heparin. *Journal of the American Medical Association* **235**: 1980–1982.

George JN (2000) Platelets. *Lancet* **355**: 1531–1539.

Gibbs NM (1957) Venous thrombosis of the lower limbs with particular reference to bed rest. *British Journal of Surgery* **5**: 209–211.

Gillespie W, Murray D, Gregg PJ *et al.* (2000) Prophylaxis against deep vein thrombosis following total hip replacement: risks and benefits of prophylaxis against venous thromboembolism in orthopaedic surgery. *Journal of Bone and Joint Surgery* **82**: 475–479.

Ginsberg KS, Liang MH, Newcomer L *et al.* (1992) Anticardiolipin antibodies and the risk for ischemic stroke and venous thrombosis. *Annals of Internal Medicine* **117**: 997–1002.

Griffin JH, Evatt B, Zimmerman TS *et al.* (1981) Deficiency of protein C in congenital thrombotic disease. *Journal of Clinical Investigation* **68**: 1370–1373.

Hamilton HW, Crawford JS, Gardiner JH *et al.* (1970) Venous thrombosis in patients with fracture of the upper end of the femur. *Journal of Bone and Joint Surgery* **52**: 268–289.

Joffe SN (1976) Deep vein thrombosis after renal transplantation. *Vascular Surgery* **10**: 134–137.

Kerr MG, Scott DB, Samuel E (1964) Studies of the inferior vena cava in late pregnancy. *British Medical Journal* **1**: 522–533.

Koster T, Rosendaal FR, de Ronde H *et al.* (1993) Venous thrombosis due to poor anticoagulant response to activated protein C: Leiden Thrombophilia Study. *Lancet* **342**: 1503–1506.

Kumar PJ (2005) *Kumar and clark clinical medicine*. WB Saunders. London.

Levi M, Ten Cate H (1999) Disseminated intravascular coagulation. *New England Journal of Medicine* **341**: 586–592.

Levine JS, Branch DW, Rauch J (2002) The antiphospholipid syndrome. *New England Journal of Medicine* **346**: 752–758.

Lim W, Crowther MA, Eikelboom JW (2006) Management of antiphospholipid antibody syndrome. *Journal of the American Medical Association* **295**: 1050–1057.

Mammen EF (1992) Pathogenesis of venous thrombosis. *Chest* **102**: 640–644S.

Mason R, Sharp D, Chuang H *et al.* (1977) The endothelium. Roles in thrombosis and haemostasis. *Archives of Pathology and Laboratory Medicine* **101**: 61–64.

May R, Thurner J (1957) The cause of the predominantly sinistral occurrence of thrombosis of the pelvic veins. *Angiology* **8**: 419–427.

Myllynen P, Kammonen M, Rokkanen P *et al.* (1985) Deep vein thrombosis and pulmonary embolism in patients with acute spinal cord injury: a comparison with nonparalyzed patients immobilized due to spinal fractures. *Journal of Trauma* **25**: 541–543.

Nicolaides AN, Kakker VV, Field ES *et al.* (1977) The origin of deep vein thrombosis: a venographic study. *British Journal of Radiology* **44**: 653–663.

Patel NH, Stookey KR, Ketcham DB *et al.* (2000) Endovascular management of acute extensive iliofemoral deep vein thrombosis caused by May–Thurner syndrome. *Journal of Vascular Interventional Radiology* **11**: 1297–1302.

Poort SR, Rosendaal FR, Reitsma PH *et al.* (1996) A common genetic variation in the 3′-untranslated region of the prothrombin gene is associated with elevated plasma prothrombin levels and an increase in venous thrombosis. *Blood* **88**: 3698–3703.

Rees MM, Rodgers GM (1993) Homocysteinemia: association of a metabolic disorder with vascular disease and thrombosis. *Thrombosis Research* **71**: 337–359.

Rossi EC, Green D, Rosen JS *et al.* (1980) Sequential changes in factor VIII and platelets preceding deep vein thrombosis in patients with spinal cord injury. *British Journal of Hematology* **45**: 143–151.

Sigel B, Ipsen J, Felix WR (1974) The epidemiology of lower extremity deep vein thrombosis in surgical patients. *Annals of Surgery* **179**: 278–290.

Stamatakis JD, Kakker VV, Sager S *et al.* (1977) Femoral vein thrombosis and total hip replacement. *British Medical Journal* **2**: 223–225.

Stead NW, Bauer KA, Kinney TR *et al.* (1983) Venous thrombosis in a family with defective release of vascular plasminogen activator and elevated plasma factor VIII, von Willebrand's factor. *American Journal of Medicine* **74**: 33–40.

Taheri SA, Williams J, Powell S, *et al.* (1987) Iliocaval compression syndrome. *American Journal of Surgery* **154**: 169–172.

Taylor FB, Toh CH, Hoots WK *et al.* (2001) Scientific subcommittee on dis-
eminated intravascular coagulation (DIC) of the International Society on
Thrombosis and Haemostasis (ISTH). Towards definition, clinical and
laboratory criteria, and a scoring system for disseminated intravascular
coagulation. *Thrombosis and Haemostasis* **86**: 1327–1330.

Thomas ML, O'dwyer JA (1977) Site of origin of deep vein thrombus in the
calf. *Acta Radiologica Diagnosis* **18**: 418–424.

Virchow R (1852) In *Gesammalte Abhandlungen zur Wissenschaftlichen Medicin*,
Anonymous (ed.). Frankfurt, Medinger Sohn und Sohn: 219–732. Cited in
VERITY (2004) Venous Thromboembolism Registry Second Annual Report.

Weitz JI, Hirsh J, Samama MM (2004) New anticoagulant drugs. *Chest* **126**:
265–286S.

Whitlon DS, Sadowski JA, Suttie JW (1978) Mechanisms of coumarin action:
significance of vitamin K epoxide reductase inhibition. *Biochemistry* **17**:
1371–1377.

Zoller B, Garcia de Frutos P, Hillarp A *et al.* (1999) Thrombophilia as a multigenic disease. *Haematologica* **84**: 59–70.

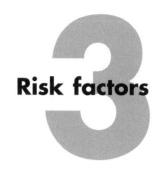

Risk factors

Overview

There are numerous reasons for people to be at an increased risk of developing a blood clot. A number of risk factors for VTE have been well defined, all of which can be traced back to an abnormality in one or more of the elements of Virchow's triad. Risk factors can now be identified in over 80% of patients presenting with VTE and typically, the more risk factors a patient has, the greater his/her risk of VTE. The risk factors, both 'strong' and 'weak', are discussed alphabetically in this chapter, and an outline on how to complete a patient risk assessment is given.

Introduction

Until the latter part of the twentieth century, VTE was considered a complication of hospitalization for major surgery, or associated with the late stage of terminal illness. Trials in the 1990s dispelled this myth by demonstrating a comparable risk for VTE in both medical and surgical hospitalized patients, as well as a high proportion of symptomatic

Venous Thromboembolism: A Nurses Guide to Prevention and Management   By Ellen Welch
© 2010 John Wiley & Sons, Ltd.

VTEs in patients who were neither hospitalized nor recovering from major illness (Anderson *et al.* 2003).

Risk factors for VTE can all be traced back to at least one of Virchow's three aetiological factors: vascular endothelial damage; stasis of blood flow; and hypercoagulability of the blood. Patients with VTE generally have at least one, if not more, risk factors (Anderson *et al.* 1992) and the risk appears to be cumulative – the more predisposing factors a patient has, the greater the risk of thrombosis (Wheeler *et al.* 1982).

The risk factors for VTE are outlined in Table 3.1. Strong risk factors (such as major general or orthopaedic surgery, spinal cord injury, major trauma, malignancy, myocardial infarction, congestive heart failure and respiratory failure) justify prophylaxis against VTE in their own right. Other recognized risk factors are associated with a lower odds ratio for the development of VTE, and are seldom enough in isolation to justify thromboprophylaxis. However, since risk factors are cumulative, a combination of two or more risk factors is usually enough to warrant VTE prophylaxis (Anderson *et al.* 2003). Practitioners should assess the strength of individual risk factors and the combined effects of all risk factors when deciding if prophylaxis is required.

Risk assessment

One of the main recommendations by the Department of Health (DH) VTE Expert Working Group, and by the 2007 NICE guidelines on reducing the risk of VTE in surgical patients, was that all hospitalized patients should receive a mandatory VTE risk assessment on admission to hospital and that they should be periodically assessed during their inpatient stay (DH 2007; NICE 2007). This allows thromboprophylaxis to be delivered according to individual need.

A universal VTE risk-scoring algorithm is yet to be published – an example of a risk assessment proforma compiled by the Department of Health is outlined in Appendix 1. All the consensus guidelines published to date agree broadly that assessment of individual risk of developing VTE should take place in all patients admitted to hospital for major trauma, major surgery or acute medical illness (SIGN 1999; DH 2007; NICE 2007).

A comprehensive assessment should include:

- Identification of personal risk factors for VTE (see Table 3.1).
- Recording any past history of VTE.
- Documenting the reason for the hospital admission.

Table 3.1 Risk factors for VTE

Age	Exponential increase in risk with age. In the general population: <40 years, annual risk 1/10000 60–69 years, annual risk 1/1000 >80 years, annual risk 1/100 (may reflect immobility and coagulation activation)
Anaesthesia/major surgery	Double the risk of VTE with general anaesthesia compared to spinal/epidural anaesthesia
Hormone therapy	Oral combined contraceptives, HRT, raloxifene, tamoxifen, 3× risk of VTE High-dose progestogens, 6× risk
Hospitalization	Acute trauma, acute illness, surgery, 10× risk
Immobility	Bed rest > 3 days, plaster cast, paralysis, 10× risk (risk increases with duration)
Obesity	Obesity (body mass index > 30 kg/m^2), 3× risk (may reflect immobility and coagulation activation)
Pregnancy/puerperium	10× risk
Previous VTE	Recurrence rate 5%/year
Prolonged travel	Increased risk in patients with established risk factors in flights over 3000 miles (see below)
Thrombophilias	Increased risk of VTE with: Low coagulation inhibitors (antithrombin, protein C or S) Activated protein C resistance (e.g. Factor V Leiden) High coagulation factors (I, II, VIII, IX, XI) Antiphospholipid syndrome High homocysteine
Other thrombotic states due to medical illness	Malignancy, 7× risk Heart failure Recent myocardial infarction/stroke Severe infection Inflammatory bowel disease Stroke Nephrotic syndrome Polycythaemia Paraproteinaemia Bechet's disease Paroxysmal nocturnal haemoglobinuria
Smoking	Moderate risk, especially in conjunction with oral contraceptives/underlying thrombophilia (Pomp *et al.* 2008)
Spinal cord injury/major trauma	High risk (combines the risks of immobility with paralysis/fractured bones)
Varicose veins	1.5× risk after major general/orthopaedic surgery Low risk after varicose vein surgery

(Adapted from SIGN 2002)

- Provision of verbal and written information of the risks of VTE and effectiveness and correct use of prophylaxis (especially in surgical patients).
- Discussion regarding avoidable risk factors, such as stopping oral contraceptive use 4 weeks prior to elective surgery.

Since VTE risk assessment is now embedded within the Clinical Negligence Scheme for Trusts (DH 2007), evidence-based risk assessment tools for VTE are required to be developed within all hospitals in the United Kingdom, and local guidelines for thromboprophylaxis should be updated for specific patient groups (see Chapter 4). A detailed breakdown of how to implement risk assessment and thromboprohylaxis is discussed further in Chapter 8.

Risk factors

Age

Incidence of VTE rises exponentially with age. Patients older than 40 years of age are at a significantly increased risk compared to younger patients, and this risk appears to double with each subsequent decade (Anderson *et al.* 2003). This may be a reflection of the accumulation of comorbidities that appear with advancing age and the tendency for older patients to be less mobile. In the MEDENOX study, age over 75 years was found to be an independent risk factor for VTE in hospitalized medical patients (Alikhan *et al.* 2004). As the population ages, the number of deaths each year due to PE is predicted to grow (Heit *et al.* 2005).

Anaesthesia and surgery

Surgery and the associated immobility and paralysis from general anaesthesia induces changes in all three elements of Virchow's triad, which accounts for its position as a strong risk factor for VTE. Vessel wall trauma and hypercoaguability occur during the procedure itself, and prolonged immobility in the postoperative period deprives the deep veins of the legs of the activity of the calf muscle pump, resulting in venous stasis. General anaesthesia decreases vascular tone and distends veins, which causes additional endothelial damage to the vessel wall. Before thromboprophylaxis was widely used, the rate of DVT in general surgical patients varied in the range 15–30%, with rates of fatal PE of 0.2–0.9% (Geerts *et al.* 2008). The current risk of thromboembolic complications is unknown because studies without prophylaxis are no longer performed, but older patients undergoing surgery with concomitant risk factors appear to be at greater risk of VTE (Geerts *et al.* 2008).

The type and duration of surgery have a clear influence on the risk of DVT, as does general perioperative care, including the state of hydration, degree of mobilization and transfusion practices (Geerts *et al.* 2008). Most patients having outpatient procedures, such as day case hernia repairs, exhibit a low frequency of DVT (Riber *et al.* 1996) and similarly the incidence of PE following cataract surgery is very low (SIGN 2002). The risk of DVT also appears to be lower following spinal/ epidural anaesthesia than after general anaesthesia in the absence of prophylaxis (Hendolin *et al.* 1981). However, the risk of perispinal hematoma may be increased with the use of prophylactic antithrombotic drugs (Horlocker *et al.* 2003); this is explored further in the next chapter.

Major general surgery

The term 'major general surgery' refers to those patients who undergo abdominal or thoracic operations requiring general anaesthesia lasting more than 30 minutes, and the risks of VTE following this have been documented extensively (SIGN 2002; Clagett *et al.* 1988).

Surgery associated with a high risk of VTE includes coronary artery bypass surgery (Josa *et al.* 1993), major urological surgery (Collins *et al.* 1988) and surgery for gynaecological malignancies (Clarke-Pearson *et al.* 1987). VTE is also common following neurosurgery (Agnelli 1999) but, given the risk of intracranial bleeding, anticoagulant therapy is seldom used (SIGN 2002). Patients undergoing major vascular surgery have a risk of VTE similar to that of patients undergoing major general surgery, and this risk is particularly high in immobilized patients with critical limb ischaemia (Libertiny & Hands 1999).

Major orthopaedic surgery, trauma and spinal cord injury

Without prophylaxis, the rate of fatality from PE following hip and knee replacement is approximately 0.4%. Considering that there are 1.25 million such procedures carried out in Europe each year, this equates to 5000 fatalities annually (House of Commons Health Committee 2005). Nearly half of these patients develop VTE; however, only 5% manifest symptoms (Anderson *et al.* 2003).

The incidence of fatal PE in trauma patients remains high, accounting for 14% of deaths following hip fracture surgery (Perez *et al.* 1995).

The problem was highlighted in 1959, when the first controlled trial of anticoagulant prophylaxis after hip fracture reduced deaths from PE from 10% to 0% (Sevitt et al. 1959). In a prospective study of 443 major trauma patients who did not receive thromboprophylaxis, the incidence of DVT was 58%, and those particularly at risk included pelvic and lower limb fractures, acute spinal cord injury, multi-system trauma and major head injuries (Geerts et al. 1994). Limited data suggest that patients with penetrating injuries have a lower risk of VTE than those patients with blunt trauma (Geerts et al. 2008).

Without prophylaxis, patients with acute spinal cord injury have the highest incidence of DVT among all hospitalized groups (SCITI 2003). Unfortunately, this group is also subject to more bleeding complications from anticoagulant therapy. The risk of PE is greatest during the first 2 weeks following injury and fatal PE is rare more than 3 months postinjury (Waring et al. 1991). Chronic paralysis following spinal cord injury is associated with atrophy of the leg muscles, which can lead to the development of small collateral vessels around old venous thrombi, which may explain these figures (Anderson et al. 2003).

Orthopaedic surgery and trauma are associated with multiple pro-thrombotic processes. Injury to bone and muscle causes extensive endothelial damage, which activates the clotting cascade, and patients are exposed to the risks of vein dilatation from anaesthetic agents, vessel trauma from the procedure and immobility following the procedure (Zaw et al. 2002).

Hormone therapy

Following the introduction of oral contraceptives containing combinations of ethinyl oestradiol and progestogen in the 1960s, there were several reports of an increasing incidence of VTE in otherwise healthy young women (Vessey et al. 1969). Despite reductions in the amounts of hormones contained in oral contraceptives since then, recent studies confirm this link, citing a four-fold increased risk in patients taking low-dose third generation oral contraceptives and a three-fold increased risk in those patients taking low-dose second generation contraceptives (Lidegaard et al. 2002).

Combined oral contraceptives induce changes in coagulation and fibrinolysis, which cause an increased tendancy to clot. It is likely that these changes have more effect in women already at an increased risk of VTE due to other risk factors, such as hereditary thrombophilic defects (van Vlijmen et al. 2007).

Women taking hormone replacement therapy (HRT) have also been shown to have a two- to fourfold increased risk of idiopathic VTE compared to those not taking HRT (Lowe et al. 2000). Men receiving oestrogen therapy for prostate cancer should also be counselled on the increased risks of VTE (Lundgren *et al.* 1986).

Hospitalization

Compared to people in the community, hospitalized patients have a more than 100fold increase in the incidence of VTE, thought to be due to their accumulation of risk factors (Heit *et al.* 2001). The impact of VTE in the surgical setting has been well studied for years, but it was only in the 1990s that VTE among hospitalized medical patients was investigated in large clinical trials. The prophylaxis in medical patients with enoxaparin (MEDENOX) study showed that approximately 15% of hospitalized medical patients who did not receive prophylaxis experienced VTE (Samama *et al.* 1999), while earlier studies reported the incidence of DVT among general medical patients to be in the range 10–26% (Cade 1982; Belch *et al.* 1981). Medical illness and surgery are both risk factors for the development of VTE and they appear to account for almost equal proportions of VTE events (22% and 24%, respectively), highlighting the need to provide prophylaxis in both groups (Heit 2008).

Hospitalization and nursing home residence combined accounts for nearly 60% of VTE events occurring in the community, and nursing home residence alone is associated with more than one-tenth of all VTE disease (Heit *et al.* 2002). Data from the Worcester DVT study carried out in the 1980s (Anderson *et al.* 1991) suggested that most episodes of VTE occur in the outpatient setting. However, studies have shown that in a group of outpatients presenting with VTE, almost half of these subjects had been hospitalized or undergone surgery in the preceding 3 months (Spencer *et al.* 2007). It has been recognized that, due to shorter hospital stays, the duration of inpatient VTE prophylaxis has decreased, and this combined with increased periods of immobilization as an outpatient means that greater emphasis should be placed on prophylaxis (Heit *et al.* 2002).

Immobility

In 1957, Gibbs observed that 15% of patients on bed rest for more than a week before death had VTE at autopsy, and this increased to 80% in patients immobilized for longer periods of time. Immobility contributes towards venous stasis and this is particularly evident in studies of paralysed patients. In a study of patients with hemiplegia, asymptomatic DVT was found in 60% of paralysed limbs of stroke patients compared with 7% in the non-paralysed limbs (Warlow *et al.* 1972). Immobility alone is a weak risk factor and does not alone provide adequate reason for prescribng prophylactic anticoagulation therapy, but prolonged immobility combined with other risk factors increases the likelihood of VTE (Anderson *et al.* 2003).

Obesity

Obesity has been recognized as an additional risk factor for VTE in patients undergoing surgery (Kakkar *et al.* 1970) and in those taking oral contraception (Vessey *et al.* 1969), but a number of studies have shown that the risk of VTE based on excess weight alone is low (Heit *et al.* 2000a; Printen *et al.* 1978). It is thought that VTE attributed to obesity may be a reflection of the immobility associated with the condition and coagulation activation (SIGN 2002).

Pregnancy and the puerperium

PE is a leading cause of maternal death following childbirth in developing countries, contributing to 20% of pregnancy-related deaths in the USA (Ronsmans C *et al.* 2006). VTE affects 100 per 100 000 pregnancies and in 30–50% of these patients, an inherited thrombophilia is present (Greer 1999). Due to the numerous risk factors to which pregnant women are exposed, the risk is three to five times higher than in the non-pregnant population (Gherman *et al.* 1999). Risk is increased by smoking, inherited thrombophilias and prior VTE (Danilenko-Dixon *et al.* 2001).

During normal pregnancy, there are profound changes in normal physiology. As well as venous stasis from blood pooling, the plasma concentrations and activities of several proteins involved in blood coagulation and fibrinolysis change, which may decrease anticoagulation and inhibit fibrinolysis, making pregnant women more susceptible to clotting (Box 3.1).

Although there are increased risks associated with pregnancy, the absolute risk of developing a clinically important VTE during this period is low (Thorogood *et al.* 1992) and the benefits of prophylactic anticoagulation is a topic for debate (Gibson PS *et al.* 2009).

If thrombosis does occur during pregnancy, anticoagulants can be used with care (Table 3.2), taking into account the increased risk of haemorrhage and other adverse events to both the mother and fetus. The adverse effects of warfarin therapy are discussed in Chapter 7. Warfarin should not be used in pregnancy in any but the highest risk situations and with informed consent, such as in women with older-generation prosthetic heart valves, in whom the thrombotic risk may outweigh the risk of the side-effects (Gibson *et al.* 2009; Bates *et al.* 2008).

Unfractionated heparin (UFH) or low molecular weight heparin (LMWH) are the treatments of choice for VTE during pregnancy and

Box 3.1 Factors causing an increased thrombotic risk during pregnancy

Increased maternal clotting factors: fibrinogen, factors VII, VIII, IX and X.

Reduced levels of protein S.

Impaired fibrinolysis due to placental fibrinolytic inhibitors.

Venous stasis and blood pooling:

- Progesterone-mediated venous dilatation.
- Compression of inferior vena cava by uterus.

Endothelial disruption of pelvic vessels: due to Caesarian section.

Acquired antithrombin deficiency: due to high proteinuric states, such as nephrotic syndrome or pre-eclampsia.

Excessive elevation of pregnancy hormones: multiple gestation/ovarian hyperstimulation syndrome.

Other maternal risk factors:

- Thrombophilia
- Family history of VTE
- Age >35
- Parity >3
- Obesity
- Immobilization
- Smoking
- Varicose veins with phlebitis
- Hyperemesis gravidarum
- Infection
- Inflammatory bowel disease
- Any condition requiring a chronic indwelling catheter

(Adapted from Gibson *et al.* 2009).

Table 3.2 Anticoagulation during pregnancy

Pregnancy risk	Recommended anticoagulation
High risk	
Current arterial or venous thromboembolism	Therapeutic LMWH or adjusted dose UFH
Prior recurrent VTE on long-term anticoagulation	Therapeutic LMWH or adjusted dose UFH
Antiphospholipid syndrome with prior VTE	Therapeutic LMWH or adjusted dose UFH ± aspirin
Mechanical heart valve	Aggressive dose therapeutic LMWH or adjusted dose UFH ± aspirin; consider warfarin between 12 and 36 weeks gestation
Moderate risk	
Single prior VTE with thrombophilia	Prophylactic LMWH or UFH
Prior idiopathic VTE, no thrombophilia	Prophylactic LMWH or UFH
Antithrombin deficiency, no VTE	Prophylactic or therapeutic LMWH or UFH
Combined thrombophilias or homozygous thrombophilic mutation, no VTE	Prophylactic LMWH or UFH
Antiphospholipid syndrome on the basis of adverse pregnancy outcomes	Prophylactic LMWH or UFH plus aspirin
Low risk	
Prior VTE with resolved temporary risk factor, no thrombophilia	Clinical surveillance or prophylactic LMWH or UFH
Single thrombophilia (other than antithrombin deficiency), no VTE	Clinical surveillance, consider aspirin
Prior adverse pregnancy outcome with thrombophilia (other than antiphospholipid syndrome), no VTE	Aspirin, consider prophylactic LMWH or UFH

(Adapted from Gibson *et al.* 2009)

should be maintained for the duration of the pregnancy and for at least 6 weeks post partum. If anticoagulation is necessary and LMWH is contraindicated, then the newer anticoagulants, such as danaparoid, fondaparinux and DTIs, can be safely considered (Gibson *et al.* 2009). The frequency of major bleeding with heparin during pregnancy is approximately 2% and is usually seen in relation to delivery (Lim *et al.* 2007). To avoid bleeding complications and the risk of epidural haematoma from regional anaesthesia used during delivery, anticoagulants are usually discontinued prior to delivery. An elective induction or Caesarean section can be scheduled at least 12 hours after a prophylactic dose of LMWH is administered or 24 hours after therapeutic LMWH (Lim *et al.* 2007).

Previous VTE

A previous history of VTE is one of the most important factors to elicit from a patient when assessing risk of further VTE. In a study of 1231 patients with VTE, 19% had at least one previous clinically recognized episode (Anderson *et al.* 1992). Heit *et al.* (2000b) found PE to be an independent predictor of reduced survival for up to three months after the initial event . As always the risk is cumulative, so when patients with previous VTE are exposed to high-risk conditions, such as major surgery or serious medical illness, they are eight times more likely to develop a new episode than patients with no history of VTE (Samama 1993).

Prolonged travel

The risk of VTE in people travelling on long-haul flights is often a subject for media attention, especially since the catchy term 'economy class syndrome' was proposed to suggest a link between the two (Symington *et al.* 1977; Cruickshank *et al.* 1988). The actual figures reported vary from study to study. Between 1977 and 1984 flight-related VTEs were associated with at least 577 deaths (25 deaths per million departures) (Sajid 2007). In 2003, Kelman *et al.* estimated the actual risk of death from flight-related VTE at 1 per 2 million passengers arriving from a flight. Clearly there is little consistent evidence to support an increasing incidence of VTE in air travellers – there is a paucity of data, with contrasting results, often based on inappropriately controlled studies or anecdotal evidence alone (SIGN 2002; Ten Wolde *et al.* 2003). What we do know, however, is that prolonged immobilization with the associated venous stasis has been recognized to increase the risk of thrombosis (Heit *et al.* 2000a), and this relationship was highlighted as far back as the Second World War. It was observed that people who had squatted motionless in bomb shelters for hours on end were more likely to die of PE (Simpson 1940). In the 1950s, similar observations were made in individuals sitting in cramped conditions during long commutes (Homans 1954).

Returning again to Virchow's familiar triad, the three factors of venous stasis, vessel-wall injury and hypercoagulability do appear to be present during air travel. The sitting position is associated with venous stasis and increased blood viscosity, and it has been demonstrated that after 1 hour there is a significant decrease in blood flow and increased concentrations of blood proteins in the legs (Landgraf *et al.* 1994; Moyses *et al.* 1987). As mentioned previously, prolonged immobility increases thrombus formation and vessel damage due to compression by aeroplane seats has also been suggested as a cause of thrombosis (Landgraf *et al.* 1994). For these reasons, even minor activity during long flights may be effective in reducing venous stasis (Noddeland *et al.* 1988).

Additional environmental factors during a flight that have been suggested to contribute to risk include dehydration due to low humidity and reduced atmospheric pressure, with consequent relative hypoxia (Bendz *et al.* 2000; Kelman *et al.* 2003; Landgraf *et al.* 1994), although evidence for these factors is lacking.

Despite the potential increase in risk in the flying environment, the average traveller does not appear to have an increased risk for symptomatic VTE (Ten Wolde *et al.* 2003), and it is still not certain that flying is any more hazardous than other activities in causing VTE – although the risk does appear to be higher in flights over 3000 miles (Lapostolle *et al.* 2001). Based on the best evidence available, the risk of symptomatic DVT after flights of more than 12 hours is 0.5% (Arya *et al.* 2002). In high-risk subjects (i.e. patients with malignancy or prone to hypercoagulability), the quantitative risk of DVT is 5% per long-haul flight and 1.6% per flight for low-risk subjects (Chee *et al.* 2005). Again, it is the risk factors listed in Table 3.1 which appear to have more of an effect on the formation of VTE than flying itself, and studies have shown that in patients with these known risk factors, VTE risk associated with flying does appear to be higher (Arya *et al.* 2002; Ansell 2001). Despite this, long-haul travel as a risk factor for VTE in its own right still remains to be proved conclusively (Hirsh *et al.* 2001). With a increase in long-haul air travel in an ageing population, it is thought that travel-related VTE may become increasingly commonplace in years to come. Airlines should work to avoid cramped seating conditions that contribute to prolonged immobility and should actively educate passengers on the dangers of VTE to encourage them to adopt preventative behaviour while aboard.

Recommendations for travellers on flights lasting 6 hours or more include:

- Adequate hydration (100–150 ml water per hour) and avoidance of alcohol.
- Avoidance of constrictive clothing.
- Frequent stretching of calf muscles for 5–10 minutes in every hour.
- Those at risk of VTE may benefit from properly fitted knee-length graduated compression stockings with ankle pressures of 14–30 mmHg. A single dose of low molecular weight heparin (1 mg/kg) has also been found to be effective in high-risk patients, but aspirin is not recommended (Geerts *et al.* 2008; Chee *et al.* 2005; Sajid *et al.* 2007).

Case study 3.1: a trip of a lifetime

A 65 year-old retired nurse visits you, asking for thromboprophy-laxis prior to a long-haul flight. She is emigrating to Australia and is concerned about the risks of VTE on the long journey there from London. Other than arthritis, your patient is well. She is an ex-smoker with no recent hospital admissions, has never had a DVT or a PE and neither has anyone in her family.

Regarding case study 3.1, how would you advise the retired nurse?

- A detailed risk assessment should be performed, as outlined in Appendix 1.
- Since she has no additional risk factors, prolonged immobility is the only major risk factor that will be a concern during the flight. Advise her that the average traveller with no VTE risk factors is at a low risk for developing VTE during the flight. She should be advised to engage in frequent stretching of the calf muscles for at least 10 minutes in every hour and to avoid constrictive clothing. Alcohol should be avoided and instead she should ensure adequate hydra-tion with plenty of water. Pharmacological prophylaxis would not be advised in her particular case, but you can fit her with knee-length graduated compression stockings to wear for the duration of the flight (see Chapter 8, Figure 8.2, p. 194).

Smoking

Tobacco smoking is a well-established risk factor for arterial events such as myocardial infarction, stroke and peripheral vascular disease; however, the evidence for smoking as an independent risk factor for VTE has been conflicting (Heit *et al.* 2000a). Previous studies have sug-gested a link (Goldhaber *et al.* 1983), whereas others have suggested that cigarette smoking has either no effect on the development of VTE (Cogo *et al.* 1994) or a 'protective effect' (Clayton *et al.* 1976). A recent large population-based case control study from The Netherlands eval-uated smoking as a risk factor and concluded that it resulted in a moderately increased risk of VTE (Pomp *et al.* 2008). When combined with use of oral contraceptives there was an eightfold higher risk, and smoking combined with the factor V Leiden mutation led to a fivefold increased risk. A high number of pack years resulted in the highest risk (Pomp *et al.* 2008).

Thrombophilia

A number of thombophilic states, such as deficiency of the natural plasma anticoagulants antithrombin, protein C and protein S, are known to contribute to the overall risk of VTE in a patient. These conditions are discussed more fully in Chapter 2.

Testing for thrombophilia should be considered in patients aged under 50 who present with recurrent VTE and in those patients with a strong family history of proven VTE [British Thoracic Society (BTS) 2003]. 25–50% of patient's with VTE will have identifiable haemostatic abnormalities on thrombophilia testing, most commonly antiphospholipid syndrome and deficiencies of antithrombin III, factor V Leiden, protein C or protein S (Greaves 2001; Seligsohn *et al.* 2001). The presence of these conditions alone rarely causes idiopathic VTE – thrombosis usually occurs with a combination of risk factors (Rosendaal 1999), e.g. if a patient with underlying factor V Leiden deficiency starts taking oestrogen therapy, the risk of VTE rises 35-fold (BTS 2003).

In practice, there are no absolute indications for clinical diagnostic thrombophilia testing and it may be carried out if there is: unprovoked or recurrent thrombosis at any age; unusual sites of thrombi, such as cerebral, mesenteric, portal or hepatic veins; thrombosis during pregnancy; hormonal medication use; or unexplained abnormalities of laboratory tests, such as a prolonged aPTT (Heit 2007). Studies have shown that although testing may be carried out frequently in patients with VTE, it does not appear to decrease the risk of recurrence (Coppens *et al.* 2007).

In pregnant patients who display an increased risk of VTE, the role of thrombophilia testing is controversial and recommendations for testing are based on the lowest quality of evidence – expert opinion (Haemostasis and Thrombosis Task Force 2001). Testing pregnant women without risk factors is not indicated, but may be performed in those with a personal or family history of VTE or known obstetric complications (Lim *et al.* 2007) (see Box 3.2).

Performing the tests are of value to:

- Understand the cause of the thromboembolic event.
- Influence the duration of therapy needed.
- Be able to offer prophylaxis to high-risk patients during periods of increased risk (e.g. orthopaedic surgery).
- Alert a patient's family to the presence of inherited risk factors.

Patients with inherited thrombophilic defects are generally given anticoagulant therapy in situations that put them at an increased risk for VTE. Prolonged or lifelong therapy with oral anticoagulants is considered even after a single thrombotic event (Zoller *et al.* 1999).

Box 3.2 How the testing is done

Blood samples should ideally be taken when the patient has not been taking any other anticoagulant for at least 10 days, otherwise this will influence the results. A full screen tests for:

- Activated protein C resistance (APCR) – factor V Leiden mutation assay should be performed when the APCR ratio is below the cut-off.
- Lupus anticoagulant testing.
- Anticardiolipin antibodies IgG and IgM.
- Antithrombin activity.
- Fasting homocysteine.
- Factor VIII activity.
- Protein C activity (perform antigen assay when activity consistently low).
- Protein S activity (perform antigen assay when activity consistently low).
- Prothrombin 20210 mutation assay.

If a patient has taken an anticoagulant within the last 10 days, the following tests can still be carried out:

- Activated protein C resistance (APCR) – factor V Leiden mutation assay should be performed when the APCR ratio is below the cut-off.
- Anticardiolipin antibodies IgG and IgM.
- Fasting homocysteine.
- Prothrombin 20210 mutation assay.

Case study 3.2: recurrent DVT

A 40 year-old lady is referred to the medical team with a right ileofemoral DVT confirmed by ultrasound. She was in hospital a week prior to this for excision of a sebaceous cyst carried out under local anaesthesia. She had a DVT in the left leg 10 years ago when she was pregnant with her son, but was only on warfarin for a short period. Her general health is good. She was adopted as a child and so is uncertain of her family history.

Regarding case study 3.2, how will you assess the lady's need for thrombophilia testing?

- Conduct a thorough risk assessment (such as the one in Appendix 1), ensuring that you enquire about all of the risk factors listed in Table 3.1.
- She doesn't have any obvious precipitating risk factors for this episode. The first episode was during pregnancy, which is a risk factor, but again, there were no other obvious precipitants. In this case, in a woman under 50, it would be wise to conduct a thrombophilia screen prior to commencing anticoagulation to establish the pathological basis of her recurrent events, so that she can be given the best treatment.
- The underlying cause of her event will determine how long she has to receive anticoagulation for. If it turns out she has an inherited thrombophilia, there will be the opportunity to offer similar testing to her family members and to educate them regarding thromboprophylaxis when they are exposed to situations that may put them at an increased risk of developing VTE.
- Routine testing is generally inappropriate and not carried out in patients with obvious risk factors. In older, hospitalized patients with no history of VTE, testing is rarely done, but in patients under 45 with unprovoked, recurrent episodes, testing should be considered.
- The testing involves a straightforward blood test, the results of which can be affected by many factors, including acute illness and certain medications. Blood should ideally be taken when the patient is not taking an anticoagulant or has not had a recent thrombotic event. In the case of an acute event, some of the blood testing can still be carried out, but only certain assays, including testing for activated protein C resistance, fasting homocysteine, anticardiolipin antibodies and the prothrombin G20210A mutation assay. Repeat testing will usually be required after completing an initial three month course of anticoagulation with warfarin (and then waiting until at least 10 days without warfarin therapy).

Thrombotic states due to medical illness

Prophylaxis in general medical patients is often overlooked, despite the fact that many medically ill patients have factors that either promote venous stasis or hypercoagulability or result in vascular damage, thus contributing to the risk of VTE (Stinnett *et al.* 2005). Hospitalization for an acute medical illness was found to be independently associated with

Table 3.3 Risk of DVT in hospitalized patients in the absence of prophylaxis

Condition	DVT prevalence (%)
General medical patients	10–20
General surgery	15–40
Major gynaecological surgery	15–40
Major urological surgery	15–40
Neurosurgery	15–40
Stroke	20–40
MI	17–34
Congestive heart failure	20–40
Medical intensive care	25–42
Hip, knee arthroplasty, hip fracture	40–60
Major trauma	40–80
Spinal cord injury	60–80

(Adapted from Spyropoulos 2005; Geerts *et al.* 2008)

an eightfold increased relative risk for VTE (Heit *et al.* 2000a). Patients with heart failure and myocardial infarction have a risk of VTE comparable to that of a moderate-risk surgical patient (Table 3.3) (Simmons *et al.* 1973). Congestive heart failure promotes venous stasis, and post-myocardial infarction (MI) patients are usually confined to bed (Anderson *et al.* 2003). Prior to the introduction of routine antithrombotic therapy, patients with acute MI had a risk of clinical PE of 2.6–9.4% and a 24% risk of asymptomatic DVT (SIGN 2002). Preventing VTE is not the primary therapeutic objective in patients with MI, but the antithrombotic treatment they receive does confer an additional benefit for the prevention of VTE.

Severe infection, inflammatory bowel disease, stroke, nephrotic syndrome, polycythaemia, paraproteinaemia, Bechet's disease and paroxysmal nocturnal haemoglobinuria have all been associated with an increased risk of VTE. Chronic inflammatory conditions and acute infections can activate endothelial cell surface receptors, leading to propagation of coagulation, resulting in a hypercoagulable state (Zaw *et al.* 2002). Patients who are immobilized in hospital due to these conditions should be candidates for thromboprophylaxis (SIGN 2002), especially if they are undergoing a surgical procedure (NICE 2007). Admission to an intensive care unit is also associated with a high risk of VTE and thromboprophylaxis should be considered (Marik *et al.* 1997). A full list of both well-established (high-risk) and probable risk factors for VTE in medical patients are listed in Box 3.3.

Box 3.3 Risk factors for VTE in hospitalized medical patients

High risk

- History of DVT or PE.
- Family history of thrombosis.
- Acute infection.
- Malignancy.
- Age > 75 years.
- Congestive heart failure.
- Stroke.
- Prolonged immobility.
- Pregnancy or postpartum.
- Acute or chronic lung disease.
- Inflammatory bowel disease.
- Shock.

Possible risk

- Paraproteinaemia.
- Behcet's disease.
- Disorders of plasminogen and plasminogen activation.
- Nephrotic syndrome.
- Polycythaemia.

- Paroxysmal nocturnal haemoglobinuria.
- Elevated serum homocysteine.
- Dysfibrinogenaemia.
- Myeloproliferative disorders.
- Age > 41 years.
- Sepsis.

Probable risk

- High-dose oestrogen therapy.
- Obesity (BMI > 25).
- Varicose veins.
- Congenital or acquired thrombophilia.
- Antithrombin deficiency.
- Positive lupus anticoagulant.
- Antiphospholipid antibodies.
- Protein S deficiency.
- Protein C deficiency.
- Positive factor V Leiden
- Elevated anticardiolipin antibodies.
- Positive prothrombin gene mutation 20210A.

(Adapted from Spyropoulos 2005)

Malignancy

The link between cancer and VTE has been well established since it was identified over 100 years ago by Trousseau (1865). The combination of VTE and malignancy is still occasionally referred to today as 'Trousseau's syndrome'. It is estimated that the annual incidence of VTE in a population of cancer patients is 1 in 200 (Lee *et al.* 2003a) and a diagnosis of cancer is associated with a 4.1-fold increased risk of thrombosis (Heit *et al.* 2000a). Autopsies reportedly show an increased rate of PE in patients with cancer (Shen *et al.* 1980) and the risk of recurrent episodes of VTE has been established to be higher in patients with an underlying malignancy (Prandoni *et al.* 2002).

There are many factors at play in the aetiology of thrombosis in patients with malignancy. Substances in the tumour cells, such as proteases and tissue factor, have procoagulant effects and the interaction between the tumour cells and macrophages lead to the activation of platelets and clotting factors, which results in the generation of thrombin (Bick 2003). Aggressive chemotherapy is associated with a 6.5 fold increased risk of thrombosis (Heit *et al.* 2000a) and this is thought to be due to vascular damage and release of tumour necrosis factor and interleukins (Bick 2003). Chemotherapy is often administered through an indwelling catheter – which further increases the risk of VTE. The thrombogenic surface of the catheters can activate platelets and cause endothelial damage, causing local activation of the coagulation cascade (Lee *et al.* 2003a; Bick 2003).

All cancer patients are at a higher risk of VTE than the general population (Falanga *et al.* 2005); however, 'mucin-producing' tumours are most strongly associated with the development of thrombosis, as suggested by autopsy studies – this includes cancers of the pancreas, lung and stomach and adenocarcinomas of unknown primary (Leiberman *et al.* 1961). The extent of the cancer also influences thrombosis risk, which may be due to concomitant antitumour therapy. 28% of patients with malignant glioma were reported to develop VTE and the risk was reported to increase throughout the course of the disease (Marras *et al.* 2000). The development of VTE in established cancer is associated with a poor prognosis (Falanga *et al.* 2005). Patients with cancer have a four- to eightfold increased risk of dying after an acute thrombotic event than patients without cancer (Prandoni *et al.* 1996).

Seemingly 'idiopathic' VTE can be a sign of occult cancer – and this is usually suspected in patients with no other apparent cause and if thrombi develop in more unusual sites, such as the upper limb, vena cavae or the portal or cerebral circulation (Lee *et al.* 2003a). Large studies have shown a 5% incidence of previously undiagnosed cancer in patients presenting with VTE (Baron *et al.* 1998). The value of extensive screening in such patients is unclear and further studies are necessary, but it is wise to consider cancer in patients presenting with VTE and to conduct routine screening through a thorough history, clinical examination and chest radiograph combined with standard laboratory tests (Fennerty 2001).

Standard anticoagulant therapy is used in patients with VTE and cancer; however, management can be problematic, due to the multiple drug interactions, frequent changes in nutritional status and alterations in liver metabolism (Falanga *et al.* 2005). The risk of bleeding complications are increased in patients with cancer (Peuscher 1981), especially postoperative bleeding. Surgery in malignant disease is also associated with a twofold higher risk of VTE than in patients without malignancy (Falanga *et al.* 2005). Long-term treatment with LMWH has been shown to decrease the risk of recurrent VTE in cancer patients as compared with heparin plus a VKA, and is associated with an improved safety profile (Lee *et al.* 2003b).

Stroke

VTE is common in patients with stroke. Patients with significant weakness and immobility are at greater risk, due to the effects of venous stasis and the general proinflammatory state which accompanies ischaemic stroke (Shorr *et al.* 2008). Studies using radiolabelled fibrinogen to identify thromboses showed that 50% of hemiplegic patients had DVTs, many of them not clinically apparent (Warlow *et al.* 1976; Cope *et al.* 1973). 13–25% of early stroke deaths can be attributed to PE, most often occurring from the second to fourth week after the onset of stroke symptoms (Kelly *et al.* 2001).

Many patients diagnosed with VTE following an ischaemic stroke have contraindications to full-intensity anticoagulation, often resulting in the use of expensive and invasive vena cava filters (Shorr *et al.* 2008). Although heparin will reduce the risk of VTE in patients with acute ischaemic stroke, evidence has shown that even low-dose heparin is associated with a significant number of symptomatic intracranial and extracranial bleeds, and routine use is not recommended (IST 1997; SIGN 1999). Aspirin given soon after the diagnosis of ischaemic stroke is confirmed improves survival and avoids one PE per 1000 patients treated (CAST 1997; IST 1997). Anticoagulant therapy (with heparin or warfarin) in acute ischaemic stroke should be reserved for patients with a high risk of VTE (previous VTE/thrombophilia) or recurrent thromboembolic stroke (e.g. mechanical heart valves, presence of atrial fibrillation), in whom the risks are judged to outweight the benefits (Sherman *et al.* 1995).

Varicose veins

Varicose veins as an independent risk factor for VTE is controversial. The presence of varicose veins has been associated with an increased risk of DVT following major surgery (Lowe *et al.* 1999); however, the risk after surgery for varicose veins appears low in the absence of other risk factors (Campbell 1996). Heit *et al.* (2000a) found that the risk of VTE associated with varicose veins decreases with age. On the balance of evidence available, varicose veins are a weak risk factor for VTE.

Conclusion

Risk factors for VTE are numerous. Certain patient groups do appear to be at a greater risk of VTE, but no patient is exempt and this chapter should illustrate why a VTE risk assessment should be considered in all patients admitted to hospital. Simply remembering that hospital admission can expose patients to an accumulation of risk factors, such as immobility, infection and invasive procedures, can prompt health professionals to implement thromboprophylactic measures, which are outlined in the next chapter.

References

Agnelli G (1999) Prevention of venous thromboembolism after neurosurgery. *Thrombosis and Haemostasis* **82**: 925–930.

Alikhan R, Cohen AT, Combe S *et al.* (2004) Risk factors for venous thromboembolism in hospitalised patients with acute medical illness: analysis of the MEDENOX study. *Archives of Internal Medicine* **164**: 963–968.

Anderson FA Jr, Wheeler HB, Goldberg RJ *et al.* (1991) A population-based perspective of the hospital incidence and case fatality rates of deep vein thrombosis and pulmonary embolism: the Worcester DVT Study. *Archives of Internal Medicine* **151**: 933–938.

Anderson FA, Wheeler HB (1992) Physician practices in the management of venous thromboembolism: a community wide survey. *Journal of Vascular Surgery* **16**: 707–714.

Anderson FA, Spencer FA (2003) Risk Factors for venous thromboembolism. *Circulation* **107**: I9–16.

Ansell JE (2001) Air travel and venous thromboembolism – is the evidence in? *New England Journal of Medicine* **345**: 828–829.

Arya R, Barnes JA, Hossain U *et al.* (2002) Long haul flights and deep vein thrombosis: a significant risk only when additional factors are also present. *British Journal of Haematology* **116**: 653–654.

Baron JA, Gridley G, Weiderpass E *et al.* (1998) Venous thromboembolism and cancer. *Lancet* **351**: 1077–1080.

Bates SM, Greer IA, Pabinger I *et al.* (2008) Venous thromboembolism, thrombophilia, antithrombotic therapy and pregnancy. *Chest* **133**: 844–886S.

Belch JJ, Lowe GD, Ward AG *et al.* (1981) Prevention of deep vein thrombosis in medical patients by low dose heparin. *Scottish Medical Journal* **26**: 115–117.

Bendz B, Rostrup M, Sevre K *et al.* (2000) Association between acute hypobaric hypoxia and activation of coagulation in human beings. *Lancet* **356**: 1657–1658.

Bick RL (2003) Cancer associated thrombosis. *New England Journal of Medicine* **349**: 109–111.

British Thoracic Society Standards of Care Committee Pulmonary Embolism Guideline Development Group (2003) British Thoracic Society guidelines for the management of suspected acute pulmonary embolism. *Thorax* **58**: 470–484.

Campbell B (1996) Thrombosis, phlebitis and varicose veins. *British Medical Journal* **312**: 198–199.

CAST (Chinese acute stroke trial) Collaborative group (1997) CAST: randomised placebo controlled trial of early aspirin use in 20 000 patients with acute ischemic stroke. *Lancet* **349**: 1641–1649.

Cade JF (1982) High risk of the critically ill for venous thromboembolism. *Critical Care Medicine* **10**: 448–450.

Chee YL, Watson HG (2005) Air travel and thrombosis. *British Journal of Haematology* **130**: 671–680.

Clagett GP, Reisch JS (1988) Prevention of venous thromboembolism in general surgical patients. Results of meta-analysis. *Annals of Surgery* **208**: 227–240.

Clarke-Pearson DL, DeLong ER, Synan IS *et al.* (1987) Variables associated with postoperative deep venous thrombosis: a prospective study of 411 gynecology patients and creation of a prognostic model. *Obstetrics and Gynecology* **69**: 146–150.

Clayton JK, Anderson JA, McNicol GP (1976) Preoperative prediction of postoperative deep vein thrombosis. *British Medical Journal* **2**: 910–912.

Cogo A, Bernardi E, Prandoni P *et al.* (1994) Acquired risk factors for deep vein thrombosis in symptomatic outpatients. *Archives of Internal Medicine* **154**: 164–168.

Collins R, Scrimgeour A, Yusuf S *et al.* (1988) Reduction in fatal pulmonary embolism and venous thrombosis by perioperative administration of subcutaneous heparin. Overview of results of randomized trials in general, orthopedic, and urologic surgery. *New England Journal of Medicine* **318**: 1162–1173.

Cope C, Tyrone MR, Skversky N (1973) Phlebographic analysis of the incidence of thrombosis in hemiplegia. *Radiology* **109**: 581–584.

Coppens M, Reinders JH, Doggen CJM *et al.* (2007) Influence of testing for inherited thrombophilia on recurrence of venous thromboembolism. *Journal of Thrombosis and Hemostasis* **5**: S2: P-M-470.

Cruickshank JM, Gorlin R, Jennett B (1988) Air travel and thrombotic episodes: the economy class syndrome. *Lancet* **2**: 497–498.

Danilenko-Dixon DR, Heit JA, Silverstein MD *et al.* (2001) Risk factors for deep vein thrombosis and pulmonary embolism during pregnancy or post partum: a population based case control study. *American Journal of Obstetrics and Gynecology* **184**: 104–110.

Department of Health (DH) (2007) *Report of the Independent Expert Working Group on the Prevention of Venous Thromboembolism in Hospitalised Patients.* Department of Health. Available at: http://www.dh.gov.uk/en/ Publicationsandstatistics/PublicationsPolicyAndGuidance/DH_073944

Falanga A, Zacharski L (2005) Deep vein thrombosis in cancer: the scale of the problem and approaches to management. *Annals of Oncology* **16**: 696–701.

Fennerty T (2001) Screening for cancer in venous thromboembolic disease. *British Medical Journal* **323**: 704–705.

Geerts WH, Code KI, Jay RM *et al.* (1994) A prospective study of venous thromboembolism after major trauma. *New England Journal of Medicine* **331**: 1601–1606.

Geerts WH, Bergqvist D, Pineo GF *et al.* (2008) Prevention of venous thromboembolism. American College of Chest Physicians evidence based clinical practice guidelines, 8th Edition. *Chest* **133**: 381–453S.

Gherman RB, Goodwin TM, Leung B *et al.* (1999) Incidence, clinical characteristics and timing of objectivly diagnosed venous thromboembolism during pregnancy. *Obstetrics and Gynecology* **94**: 730–734.

Gibbs NM (1957) Venous thrombosis of the lower limbs with particular reference to bedrest. *British Journal of Surgery* **45**: 209–236.

Gibson PS, Powrie R (2009) Anticoagulants and pregnancy: when are they safe? *Cleveland Clinic Journal of Medicine* **762**: 113–127.

Goldhaber SZ, Savage DD, Garrison RJ *et al.* (1983) Risk factors for pulmonary embolism: the Framingham study. *American Journal of Medicine* **74**: 1023–1028.

Greaves M (2001) Thrombophilia. *Clinical Medicine* **1**: 432–435.

Greer IA (1999) Thrombosis in pregnancy: maternal and fetal issues. *Lancet* **353**: 1258–1265.

Haemostasis and Thrombosis Task Force, British Committee for Standards in Haematology. Investigation and management of heritable thrombophilia (2001). *British Journal of Haematology* **114**: 512–528.

Heit JA, Silverstein MD, Mohr DN *et al.* (2000a) Risk factors for deep vein thrombosis and pulmonary embolism: a population based case control study. *Archives of Internal Medicine* **160**: 809–815.

Heit JA, Silverstein MD, Mohr DN *et al.* (2000b) Predictors for recurrence after deep vein thrombosis and pulmonary embolism: a population based cohort study. *Archives of Internal Medicine* **160**: 761–768.

Heit JA, Melton LJ 3rd, Lohse CM *et al.* (2001) Incidence of venous thromboembolism in hospitalized patients versus community residents. *Mayo Clinic Proceedings* **76**: 1102–1110.

Heit JA, O'Fallon WM, Petterson TM *et al.* (2002) Relative impact of risk factors for deep vein thrombosis and pulmonary embolism. A population based study. *Archives of Internal Medicine* **162**: 1245–1248.

Heit JA (2005) Venous thromboembolism, disease burden, outcomes and risk factors. State of the art. *Journal of Thrombosis and Haemostasis* **3**: 1611–1617.

Heit JA (2007) Thrombophilia: common questions on laboratory assessment and management. *Hematology* **1**: 127–135.

Heit JA (2008) Venous thromboembolism: mechanisms, treatment and public awareness. The epidemiology of venous thromboembolism in the community. *Arteriosclerosis, Thrombosis, and Vascular Biology* **28**: 370–372.

Hendolin H, Mattila MAK, Poikolainen E (1981) The effect of lumbar epidural analgesia on the development of deep vein thrombosis of the legs after open prostatectomy. *Acta Chirurgica Scandinavica* **147**: 425–429.

Hirsh J, O'Donnell MJ (2001) Venous thromboembolism after long flights: are airlines to blame? *Lancet* **357**, 1461–1462.

Homans J (1954) Thrombosis of the leg veins due to prolonged sitting. *New England Journal of Medicine* **250**: 148–149.

Horlocker TT, Wedel DJ, Benzon H *et al.* (2003) Regional anesthesia in the anticoagulated patient: defining the risks (the Second ASRA Consensus Conference on Neuraxial Anesthesia and Anticoagulation). *Regional Anesthesia and Pain Medicine* **28**: 172–197.

House of Commons Health Committee (2005) *The Prevention of Venous Thromboembolism in Hospitalised Patients.* HC99. Stationery Office, London. Available at: www.publications.parliament.uk/pa/cm200405/cmselect/cmhealth/99/9902.htm*evidence_downloaded_29

International Stroke Trial Collaborative Group (IST) (1997) The International Stroke Trial. A randomised trial of aspirin, subcutaneous heparin, both or neither among 19,435 patients with acute ischemic stroke. *Lancet* **349**: 1569–1581.

Josa M, Siouffi SY, Silverman AB *et al.* (1993) Pulmonary embolism after cardiac surgery. *Journal of the American College of Cardiology* **21**: 990–996.

Kakkar VV, Howe CT, Nicolaides AN *et al.* (1970) Deep vein thrombosis of the leg: is there a 'high risk' group? *American Journal of Surgery* **120**: 527–530.

Kelly J, Rudd A, Lewis R *et al.* (2001) Venous thromboembolism after acute stroke. *Stroke* **32**: 262–267.

Kelman CW, Kortt MA, Becker NG *et al.* (2003) Deep vein thrombosis and air travel: record linkage study. *British Medical Journal* **327**: 1072.

Landgraf H, Vanselow B, Schulte-Huermann D *et al.* (1994) Economy class syndrome: rheology, fluid balance and lower leg edema during a simulated 12 hour long distance flight. *Aviation, Space and Environmental Medicine* **65**: 930–935.

Lapostolle F, Surget V, Borron SW *et al.* (2001) Severe pulmonary embolism associated with air travel. *New England Journal of Medicine* **345**: 828–829.

Lee AYY, Levine MN (2003a) Venous thromboembolism and cancer: risks and outcomes. *Circulation* **107**: 17–21.

Lee AYY, Levine MN, Baker RI *et al.* (2003b) Low-molecular-weight heparin versus a coumarin for the prevention of recurrent venous thromboembolism in patients with cancer. *New England Journal of Medicine* **349**: 146–153.

Leiberman JS, Borrero J, Urdanetam E *et al.* (1961) Thrombophlebitis and cancer. *Journal of the American Medical Association* **177**: 542–545.

Libertiny G, Hands L (1999) Deep venous thrombosis in peripheral vascular disease. *British Journal of Surgery* **86**: 907–910.

Lidegaard O, Edstom B, Kreiner S (2002) Oral contraceptives and venous thromboembolism: a five year national case control study. *Contraception* **65**: 187–196.

Lim W, Eikelboom JW Ginsberg JS (2007) Inherited thrombophilia and pregnancy associated venous thromboembolism. *British Medical Journal* **334**: 1318–1321.

Lowe GD, Haverkate F, Thompson SG *et al.* (1999) Prediction of deep vein thrombosis after elective hip replacement surgery by preoperative clinical and haemostatic variables: the ECAT DVT Study. European Concerted Action on Thrombosis. *Thrombosis and Haemostasis* **81**: 879–886.

Lowe G, Woodward M, Vessey M *et al.* (2000) Thrombotic variables and risk of idiopathic venous thromboembolism in women aged 45–64 years. Relationship to hormone replacement therapy. *Thrombosis and Haemostasis* **83**: 530–535.

Lundgren R, Sundin T, Colleen S *et al.* (1986) Cardiovascular complications of estrogen therapy for nondisseminated prostatic carcinoma. A preliminary report from a randomized multicenter study. *Scandanavian Journal of Urology and Nephrology* **20**: 101–105.

Marik PE, Andrews L, Maini B (1997) The incidence of deep venous thrombosis in ICU patients. *Chest* **111**: 661–664.

Marras LC, Geerts WH, Perry JR (2000) The risk of venous thromboembolism is increased throughout the course of malignant glioma: an evidence based review. *Cancer* **89**: 640–646.

Moyses C, Cederholm-Williams SA, Michel CC (1987) Haemoconcentration and accumulation of white cells in the feet during venous stasis. *International Journal of Microcirculation, Clinical and Experimental* **5**: 311–320.

National Institute for Clinical Excellence (NICE) (2007) Venous thromboembolism. Reducing the risk of venous thromboembolism (deep vein thrombosis and pulmonary embolism) in inpatients undergoing surgery. NICE Clinical Guideline No. 46. Available at: www.nice.org.uk/CG046

Noddeland H, Winkel J (1988) Effects of leg activity and ambient barometric pressure on foot swelling and lower limb skin temperature during 8 h of sitting. *European Journal of Applied Physiology and Occupational Physiology* **57**: 409–414.

Perez JV, Warwick DJ, Case CP *et al.* (1995) Death after proximal femoral fracture: an autopsy study. *Injury* **26**: 237–240.

Peuscher FW (1981) Thrombosis and bleeding in cancer patients. *Netherlands Journal of Medicine* **24**: 23–35.

Pomp ER, Rosendaal FR, Doggen CJM (2008) Smoking increases the risk of venous thrombosis and acts synergistically with oral contraceptive use. *American Journal of Hematology* **83**: 97–102.

Prandoni P Lensing AWA, Cogo A *et al.* (1996) The long-term clinical course of acute deep venous thrombosis. *Annals of Internal Medicine* **125**: 1–7.

Prandoni P, Lensing AW, Piccioli A *et al.* (2002) Recurrent venous thromboembolism and bleeding complications during anticoagulant treatment in patients with cancer and venous thrombosis. *Blood* **100**: 3484–3488.

Printen KJ, Miller EV, Mason EE *et al.* (1978) Venous thromboembolism in the morbidly obese. *Surgery, Gynecology and Obstetrics* **147**: 63–64.

Riber C, Alstrup N, Nymann T *et al.* (1996) Postoperative thromboembolism after day case herniorrhaphy. *British Journal of Surgery* **83**: 420–421.

Ronsmans C, Graham WJ (2006) Maternal mortality: who, when, where and why. *Lancet* **368**: 1189–1200.

Rosendaal FR (1999) Venous thrombosis: a multicausal disease. *Lancet* **353**: 1167–1173.

Sajid MS, Iftikhar M, Rimple J *et al.* (2007) Literature review of deep vein thrombosis in air travellers. *International Journal of Surgery* **10**: 1–10.

Samama MM (1993) Epidemiology of risk factors of deep vein thrombosis (DVT) of the lower limbs in community practice: the SIRIUnited States study. *Thrombosis and Haemostasis* **69**: 763–768.

Samama MM, Cohen AT, Darmon JY *et al.* (1999) A comparison of enoxaparin with placebo for the prevention of venous thromboembolism in acutely ill medical patients: Prophylaxis in Medical Patients with Enoxaparin Study Group. *New England Journal of Medicine* **341**: 793–800.

Scottish Intercollegiate Guidelines Network (SIGN) (1999) National Clinical Guidelines on Antithrombotic Therapy. University of Dundee. Available at: http://www.sign.ac.uk/pdf/sign36.pdf

Scottish Intercollegiate Guidelines Network (SIGN) (2002) National Clinical Guidelines on Prophylaxis of Venous Thromboembolism. University of Dundee. Available at: http://www.sign.ac.uk/pdf/sign62.pdf

Seligsohn U, Lubetsky A (2001) Genetic susceptibility to venous thrombosis. *New England Journal of Medicine* **344**: 1222–1231.

Sevitt S, Gallagher NG (1959) Prevention of venous thrombosis and pulmonary embolism in injured patients: a trial of anticoagulant prophylaxis with phenindione in middle aged and elderly patients with fractured necks of femurs. *Lancet* **2**: 981–989.

Shen VS, Pollak EW (1980) Fatal pulmonary embolism in cancer patients: is heparin prophylaxis justified? *South Medical Journal* **73**: 841–843.

Sherman DG, Dyken ML, Gent M *et al.* (1995) Antithrombotic therapy for cerebrovascular disorders. An update. *Chest* **108**: 444–456S.

Shorr AF, Jackson WL, Sherner JH *et al.* (2008) Differences between low molecular weight and unfractionated heparin for venous thromboembolism prevention following ischemic stroke. *Chest* **133**: 149–155.

Simmons AV, Sheppard MA, Cox AF (1973) Deep venous thrombosis after myocardial infarction. *Lancet* **35**: 623–625.

Simpson K (1940) Shelter deaths from pulmonary embolism. *Lancet* **2**: 744.

Spencer FA, Lessard D, Emery C *et al.* (2007) Venous thromboembolism in the outpatient setting. *Archives of Internal Medicine* **167**: 1471–1475.

Spinal Cord Injury Thromboprophylaxis Investigators (SCITI) (2003) Prevention of venous thromboembolism in the acute treatment phase after spinal cord injury: a randomized multicenter trial comparing low-dose heparin plus intermittent pneumatic compression with enoxaparin. *Journal of Trauma* **54**: 1116–1126.

Spyropoulos AC (2005) Emerging strategies in the prevention of venous thromboembolism in hospitalised medical patients. *Chest* **128**: 958–969.

Stinnett JM, Pendleton R, Skordos L *et al.* (2005) Venous thromboembolism prophylaxis in medically ill patients and the development of strategies to improve prophylaxis rates. *American Journal of Hematology* **78**: 167–170.

Symington IS, Stack BH (1977) Pulmonary thromboembolism after travel. *British Journal of Diseases of the Chest* **71**: 138–140.

Ten Wolde MT, Kraaijenhagen RA, Schiereck J *et al.* (2003) Travel and the risk of symptomatic venous thromboembolism. *Thrombosis and Haemostasis* **89**: 499–505.

Thorogood M, Mann J, Murphy M *et al.* (1992) Risk factors for fatal venous thromboembolism in young women: a case control study. *International Journal of Epidemiology* **21**: 48–52.

Trousseau A (1865) Phlegmasia alba dolens. In *Clinique Médicale de l'Hôtel-Dieu de Paris*, Vol **3**. Ballière, Paris: 654–712.

Van Vlijmen EFW, Brouwer JP, Veeger NJGM *et al.* (2007) Oral contraceptives and the absolute risk of venous thromboembolism in women with single or multiple thrombophilic defects. *Archives of Internal Medicine* **167**: 282–289.

Vessey MP, Doll R (1969) Investigation of relation between use of oral contraceptives and thromboembolic disease: a further report. *British Medical Journal* **2**: 651–657.

Waring WP, Karunas RS (1991) Acute spinal cord injuries and the incidence of clinically occuring thromboembolic disease. *Paraplegia* **29**: 8–16.

Warlow C, Ogston D, Douglas AS (1972) Venous thrombosis following strokes. *Lancet* **1**: 1305–1306.

Warlow C, Ogston D, Douglas AS (1976) Deep venous thrombosis of the legs after strokes. Part 1. Incidence and predisposing factors. *BMJ* **1**: 1178–1181.

Wheeler HB, Anderson FA, Cardullo PA *et al.* (1982) Suspected deep vein thrombosis. Management by impedence plethysmography. *Archives of Surgery* **117**: 1206–1209.

Zaw HM, Osborne IC, Pettit PN *et al.* (2002) Risk factors for venous thromboembolism in orthopedic surgery. *Israel Medical Association Journal* **4**: 1040–1042.

Zoller B, Garcia de Frutos P, Hillarp A *et al.* (1999) Thrombophilia as a multigenic disease. *Haematologica* **84**: 59–70.

Prophylaxis

Overview

The Department of Health (DH) has recognized VTE as a major cause of mortality and morbidity in hospitalized patients. The House of Commons Health Select Committee published a report in 2005 which highlighted the scale of the problem, with emphasis on the fact that the majority of deaths from VTE are preventable with correct education and appropriate use of thromboprophylaxis (HCHC 2005). This chapter presents the evidence for prevention and examines the longer-term consequences of VTE in those patients who survive an acute episode, including post-thrombotic syndrome (PTS) and recurrent VTE. Mechanical and pharmacological methods of prophylaxis appropriate to specific patient risk groups are discussed.

Evidence for prevention

Hundreds of randomized trials and more than 25 evidence-based guidelines on the benefits and safety of thromboprophylaxis have been published since 1986 (Geerts *et al.* 2008). In the United Kingdom alone,

Venous Thromboembolism: A Nurses Guide to Prevention and Management   By Ellen Welch
© 2010 John Wiley & Sons, Ltd.

the prevention of VTE has become a priority and multiple organizations have established guidelines and advice on the subject (see Appendix 2). An independent VTE expert working group has been established to generate guidance on how thromboprophylaxis can be implemented in the United Kingdom (DH 2007), and the National Institute for Health and Clinical Excellence (NICE) have issued guidelines on reducing the risk of VTE in surgical patients (NICE 2007) and are currently working on similar guidelines for medical patients. The main rationale for thromboprophylaxis is listed in Table 4.1. As always, healthcare professionals should exercise their clinical judgement when making decisions regarding the appropriateness of VTE prophylaxis, using evidence-based data to guide them.

If the mortality figures and statistics presented in the preceding chapters are not enough evidence to convincingly sell the argument for thromboprophylaxis, then let's look at the long-term consequences of thrombosis in those patients who survive an acute episode.

Table 4.1 Rationale for thromboprophylaxis in hospitalized patients

Rationale	Description
High prevalence of VTE	Most hospitalized patients have VTE risk factors
	DVT is common in many hospitalized patient groups
	Hospital-acquired VTE is usually clinically silent
	Difficult to predict which at-risk patients will develop symptomatic complications
	Screening at-risk patients is neither effective nor cost-effective
Adverse consequences of unprevented VTE	Symptomatic DVT and PE
	Fatal PE
	Costs of investigating symptomatic patients
	Risks and costs of treating unprevented VTE
	Increased future risk of recurrent VTE
	Chronic post-thrombotic syndrome
Efficacy and effectiveness of thromboprophylaxis	Thromboprophylaxis is highly efficacious at preventing DVT
	Thromboprophylaxis is highly efficacious at preventing symptomatic VTE and fatal PE
	Prevention of DVT also prevents PE
	Cost effectiveness of prophylaxis has been repeatedly demonstrated

(Adapted from Geerts *et al.* 2008)

Post-thrombotic syndrome (PTS)

Clinical features and pathophysiology

Deep vein thrombosis (DVT) damages the deep venous valves, leading to venous reflux and venous hypertension, and consequently reduces venous return in the affected limb. When this reduced circulation leads to pain, heaviness, pruritis and swelling of the leg, it is known as the post-thrombotic syndrome (Kearon 2003). As it increases in severity, the increased pressure causes oedema, rupture of small superficial veins and deposition of haemosiderin, resulting in skin hyperpigmentation and varicose eczema. Subsequent subcutaneous fibrosis and atrophy leads to further skin changes, including lipodermatosclerosis and chronic skin ulceration (Hopkins *et al.* 1992). Table 4.2 outlines the clinical features of PTS.

Diagnosis

The diagnosis of PTS is largely clinical, since ultrasound results can be difficult to interpret due to persistent abnormalities after the initial DVT (Kahn *et al.* 2004). The severity of PTS can be assessed using clinical scales such as the Villalta scale, which grades severity from 0 to 3, based on the presence of typical symptoms and signs (Villalta *et al.* 1994). The Ginsberg scale appears to be more effective at identifying severe disease and defines PTS as the presence of daily leg pain and swelling for 1 month, occurring for 6 months or more after DVT, made worse by standing/walking and relieved by rest/leg elevation (Kahn *et al.* 2006). There appears to be little correlation between the severity

Table 4.2 Clinical features of PTS

Symptoms	Signs
Heaviness	Oedema
Pain	Telangiectasia
Swelling	Venous ectasia
Itching	Varicose veins
Cramps	Venous dilatation
Paraesthesia	Hyperpigmentation
Bursting pain	Stasis dermatitis (eczema)
	Redness
Symptoms worse on activity/prolonged standing and improved by rest/recumbency	Dependent cyanosis
	Lipodermatosclerosis
	Healed or open ulcer

(Adapted from Kahn *et al.* 2004)

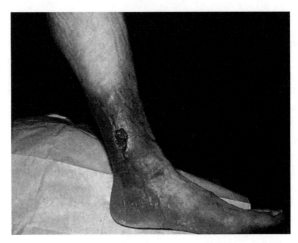

Figure 4.1 Chronic leg ulceration. Included with the permission of the King's Thrombosis Centre (www.kingsthrombosiscentre.org.uk/library.php).

of the initial DVT and the development of PTS (Prandoni *et al.* 1996), and factors predictive of PTS include female sex, increasing age, hormone therapy, varicose veins, abdominal surgery and obesity (Kahn *et al.* 2004).

Consequences and costs
PTS develops in up to 50% of patients within 1–2 years of DVT; among these, 25% suffer with severe PTS (Kahn *et al.* 2002a). Once PTS is established, patients can progress to develop stasis ulcers and may suffer recurrent inflammatory episodes and both fungal and bacterial infections. This recurrent inflammation can worsen venous damage, resulting in disfigurement and an elevated risk of DVT. Patients with PTS are often immobile, resulting in a decreased quality of life and an increased societal burden (Kahn *et al.* 2002b). Around 100 000 people in England and Wales are thought to suffer with venous leg ulcers (Figure 4.1) as a consequence of DVT and the cost of treating these chronic complications of DVT is thought to exceed £400 million each year in the United Kingdom (HCHC 2005). Similar figures are cited from the United States and it is estimated that 2 million work days are lost annually due to leg ulcers (Phillips *et al.* 1994).

Management
Treatments for PTS are limited and the overwhelming message is to focus on the prevention of DVT in high-risk patient groups (Geerts *et al.* 2008). Management of established PTS and venous ulceration

focuses on limb elevation, lymphatic massage, exercise, skin care and compression therapy (Kahn *et al.* 2004). Compression stockings may reduce limb swelling in some patients with PTS, and severe PTS can be improved with long-term use of an intermittent compression extremity pump (Kearon *et al.* 2003). Pentoxifylline (400 mg orally three times daily), a drug proved to promote blood flow, has been recommended by the American College of Chest Physicians (ACCP) for patients with venous leg ulcers in addition to local care and compression (Kearon *et al.* 2008). In patients with persistent venous ulcer, rutosides (compounds derived from horse chestnut to treat oedema formation) can be administered alongside skin care and compression therapy (Kearon *et al.* 2008).

The best available treatment remains prevention. Once DVT is established, anticoagulation and compression are required to prevent recurrent VTE and PTS.

Recurrent VTE
The risk of recurrent VTE depends on whether or not patients have continuing risk factors, as discussed in the previous chapter. Without anticoagulation, about half the patients with symptomatic VTE will experience a recurrence within three months (Kearon 2003). Even with anticoagulation, patients with transient risk factors have a 3% per year risk of recurrence , and those with a continuing risk factor have at least a 10% per year risk (Kearon 2003). Recurrent episodes of VTE tend to duplicate the initial mode of presentation and the risk of fatal PE is threefold higher after an episode of PE than of DVT (Heit *et al.* 1999; Kearon 2003). Preventing VTE from the outset avoids patients being faced with the persistent fear that VTE is going to strike again – and worrying that maybe the next episode will be fatal.

Complications of PE
Approximately 10% of symptomatic PEs are rapidly fatal (Stein *et al.* 1995) and about one-quarter of patients with PE die within 1 year (Kearon 2003). The many complications of PE are listed in Box 4.1; however, chronic pulmonary hypertension is associated with serious morbidity and mortality (Pengo *et al.* 2004). Pulmonary hypertension (chronically elevated blood pressure in the pulmonary circulation) occurs as a complication of PE in 3–4% of patients who survive the initial episode (Pengo *et al.* 2004). Patients complain of progressive shortness of breath, exercise intolerance and, later, exertional chest pain and syncope may occur. Without intervention (with pulmonary thromboendarterectomy) the rate of survival is low, and is proportional to the degree of pulmonary hypertension present (Fedullo *et al.* 2001).

Box 4.1 Complications of PE

- Pulmonary hypertension.
- Sudden cardiac death.
- Pulseless electrical activity.
- Cardiac arrhythmias.
- Cor pulmonale.
- Severe hypoxaemia.
- Right to left intracardiac shunt.
- Lung infarction.
- Pleural effusion.
- Paradoxical embolism.

Yet again, prevention is the key to preventing such morbidity and mortality.

Methods of prophylaxis

> The whole issue of thromboprophylaxis needs to be raised within medical schools so that junior doctors try to implement this from the first day of their postgraduate working lives.
>
> *(Acute NHS Trust. All Party Parliamentary Thrombosis Group Annual Audit Report)*

The two main methods of prophylaxis against VTE involve mechanical methods (such as graduated compression stockings and intermittent pneumatic compression devices) and pharmacological methods (using anticoagulants such as unfractionated heparin and low molecular weight heparin). Virchow's triad states that the three predisposing factors of venous stasis, vessel wall trauma and hypercoagulability all contribute to the formation of a clot. Prophylactic measures aim to target as many components of the triad as possible. Mechanical methods focus mainly on venous stasis, preventing this by increasing venous outflow within the leg veins. If venous stasis is prevented, this also can reduce tearing of the endothelium of the blood vessels (see Chapter 8). Pharmacological methods deal with the 'hypercoagulability' aspect of the triad and attempts to alter the substances in the blood responsible for clotting (see Chapter 7).

General measures should also be endorsed, such as early mobilization and leg exercises to reduce the venous stasis brought about by prolonged immobilization. In patients who are unable to mobilize, then adequate hydration should be ensured (SIGN 1999).

Mechanical prophylaxis

In 1956, Wright *et al.* used a radioisotope clearance technique which showed that the velocity of venous flow was reduced in limbs that were horizontal at rest and increased with elevation or movement. This provided a rationale for the practice of early ambulation after operation (Canavarro 1946) and the wearing of elastic stockings (Wilkins and Stanton 1953). Graduated compression stockings (GCS), intermittent pneumatic compression (IPC) devices and venous foot pumps (VFPs) have all been shown to reduce the risk of DVT in a number of patient groups, although they are generally less effective and not as well researched as the pharmacological methods of prophylaxis (Geerts *et al.* 2008). They act by increasing venous outflow, thereby reducing venous stasis within the leg veins. One of their biggest advantages is the avoidance of bleeding complications that can occur with anticoagulation, and they are primarily recommended in patients at high risk of bleeding, or as an adjunct to anticoagulant-based prophylaxis (Geerts *et al.* 2008).

One of the main advantages of these mechanical methods is the reduction in the risk of PTS – from 49% to 26%, according to one study (Prandoni *et al.* 2004). However, they need to be used in caution in patients with problems such as peripheral arterial insufficiency (Geerts *et al.* 2008).

Mechanical methods of prophylaxis are described in further detail in Chapter 8.

Pharmacological prophylaxis

The pharmacology of the agents licensed for prophylaxis of VTE listed below are covered in greater detail in Chapter 7.

Unfractionated heparin (UFH) and low molecular weight heparin (LMWH)

A meta-analysis carried out by Mismetti *et al.* (2000) showed that UFH and LMWH are equally effective at reducing the incidence of VTE, but LMWH is safer, with a 52% lower risk of bleeding. Two major randomized control trials, the MEDENOX (Samama *et al.* 1999) and PREVENT (Leizorovicz *et al.* 2004a) trials, investigated the efficacy of LMWH and both found the incidence of DVTs to be reduced.

Numerous trials have shown UFH and LMWH to have a similar efficacy and bleeding rate; however, the side-effect profile of LMWH is more favourable than that of UFH and LMWH allows a once-daily dosing regimen without the need for monitoring (Geerts *et al.* 2008). Table 7.9 on page 182 outlines the advantages of LWMH over UFH.

Fondaparinux

The synthetic pentasaccharide fondaparinux has been shown to be more effective than LMWH in the reduction of asymptomatic DVT in orthopaedic patients, although not in the reduction of symptomatic DVT, PE or mortality (Bounameaux *et al.* 2002). It has been approved for VTE prophylaxis in patients undergoing surgery for hip fracture and hip or knee joint replacement. However, the cost of treatment with fondaparinux has been estimated at approximately $44 per day in comparison to $3 per day with UFH treatment and $35 per day with LMWH treatment (Anonymous 2002).

Danaparoid is a mixture of low molecular weight sulphated glycosaminoglycans and acts in a similar way to heparin and fondaparinux, with anti-Xa activity. It is normally used when the patient has had heparin-induced thrombocytopenia (HIT), since the antibody against heparin does not cross-react with it (NICE 2007).

Vitamin K antagonists (VKAs)

Warfarin is effective in the prophylaxis of asymptomatic DVT, but is not widely used for this indication in the United Kingdom – mainly due to the increased bleeding risk associated with its use and because of the need for daily monitoring (SIGN 1999; Geerts *et al.* 2008). VKAs were effective in reducing DVT and clinical PE compared to placebo in orthopaedic patients, but less effective than LMWH (Mismetti *et al.* 2004). In patients already on long-term VKA therapy, for example for prosthetic heart valves, who become immobilized by illness or surgery, continued use may be appropriate in the prophylaxis of VTE. However, if bleeding risk becomes a concern, such as before surgery, it may be necessary to replace VKA therapy with either UFH or LMWH and mechanical prophylaxis (SIGN 2002).

Aspirin

Antiplatelet drugs are highly effective at reducing major vascular events in patients with atherosclerotic disease, but the use of aspirin for preventing VTE is controversial. SIGN (2002) advocates the use of aspirin, based mainly on one large trial showing a reduction in symptomatic DVT and fatal PE with aspirin prophylaxis, with only a small increased risk of minor bleeding (PEP 2000). However, (Geerts WH *et al.* 2008) advise against aspirin use in view of the increased risk of bleeding, especially if combined with other antithrombotic agents. They cite a number of trials displaying no significant benefit from aspirin therapy, and found that aspirin is inferior to other established prophylactic modalities, such as LMWH (Geerts *et al.* 2008).

Consensus guideline recommendations

> Our most important recommendation is that thrombosis committees and thrombosis teams should be established in each hospital to promote best practice now.
>
> *(House of Commons Health Select Committee 2005)*

The approach of the ACCP in their guidelines on the prevention of VTE is to target specific groups of patients identified at being at risk of thromboembolism, and similar guidelines by organizations such as the Scottish Intercollegiate Guidelines Network (SIGN) follow suit. Such guidelines aim to assist individual hospitals, general practitioners and health boards to produce their own local guidelines to identify patients at risk of VTE and, after assessing the balance of bleeding risks, to initiate effective and timely prophylaxis.

Decisions regarding initiation of prophylaxis should be made based on specific knowledge of each patient's risk factors for VTE, the potential for adverse consequences with prophylaxis and the options available at your specific institution. Care should be taken in patients with renal failure, for example – a reduced creatinine clearance can lead to accumulation of several anticoagulants, resulting in an increased risk of bleeding (Geerts *et al.* 2008). Similarly, care should be taken when using anticoagulants in patients undergoing spinal or epidural anaesthesia, in view of the increased risk of perispinal haematoma, which can lead to spinal cord ischaemia and subsequent paraplegia (Geerts *et al.* 2008). The current recommendations for the 'at risk' groups are outlined below.

Surgical patients

The type of surgery being performed determines the risk of VTE as well as the risk of bleeding, therefore it is useful to consider thromboprophylaxis for the different surgical specialities separately. It may be useful to stratify patients undergoing general surgery into risk categories to allow the most appropriate prophylaxis to be used (see Box 4.2).

Box 4.2 Risk of VTE in surgical patients

Low risk   Minor procedure in patients aged <40 years, with minimal immobility postoperatively and no risk factors for VTE (see Table 3.1, p. 43)

Moderate risk   Any surgery in patients aged 40–60 years

Major surgery in patients aged <40 years and with no other risk factors for VTE

Minor surgery in patients with one of more risk factors for VTE

High risk   Major surgery in patients aged over 60 years

Major surgery in patients aged 40–60 years with one or more risk factors

Very high risk   Major surgery in patients aged > 40 years with previous VTE, cancer or known hypercoagulable state

Major orthopaedic surgery

Elective neurosurgery

Multiple trauma or acute spinal cord injury

(Blann *et al.* 2006) reproduced with permission from the BMJ group

---

There are general guidelines that are relevant regardless of the surgical specialty (NICE 2007):

- Patients should be informed of the risks of VTE and how to prevent it.
- All inpatients undergoing surgery should be offered correctly fitted thigh-length graduated compression stockings (unless contraindicated), which they should be encouraged to wear until they return to their usual level of mobility.
- Patients with individual risk factors for VTE (see Table 3.1, p. 43) should be offered LMWH.
- Vena cava filters should be considered for surgical inpatients with recent (within one month) or existing VTE and a contraindication to coagulation.
- The risks and benefits of stopping established anticoagulation or antiplatelet therapy should be assessed.
- Since regional anaesthesia reduces the risk of VTE compared with general anaesthesia, options should be discussed with the patient. If regional anaesthesia is used, pharmacological prophylaxis should be timed carefully to minimize the risk of haematoma.
- Postoperatively, early mobilization should be encouraged, alongside leg exercises and adequate hydration.

Orthopaedic surgery

Major elective or traumatic orthopaedic surgery is high risk for the development of VTE and use of thromboprophylaxis within the specialty has been routine for more than 15 years (SIGN 2002; NICE 2007; Geerts *et al.* 2008). Major orthopaedic surgery includes hip and knee arthroplasty and hip fracture repair. Current guidelines from NICE advise:

> Mechanical prophylaxis combined with either LMWH or fondaparinux. This should be continued for four weeks following hip fracture surgery, and in those patients with one or more risk factor for VTE.
>
> *(NICE 2007)*

General surgery

The term 'major general surgery' refers to those patients who undergo abdominal or thoracic operations requiring general anaesthesia lasting more than 30 minutes (SIGN 2002):

- Low-risk general surgical patients (see Box 4.2) are advised to use mechanical prophylaxis only.
- Moderate-risk general surgical patients (see Box 4.2) should receive prophylactic LMWH or UFH.
- High-risk general surgical patients (see Box 4.2) should also receive prophylactic LMWH or UFH combined with GCS and continue prophylactic LMWH following hospital discharge (Geerts *et al.* 2008).

Vascular surgery

- Patients should be offered mechanical prophylaxis.
- Patients with one or more risk factor for VTE should also be offered LMWH (NICE 2007) or UFH (Geerts *et al.* 2008).

Gynaecological surgery (excluding Caesarean section)

- Patients should be offered mechanical prophylaxis.
- Patients with one or more risk factors for VTE should also be offered LMWH (NICE 2007) or UFH (Geerts *et al.* 2008).
- High-risk patients (such as those with cancer or previous VTE) should continue LMWH prophylaxis for 2–4 weeks following hospital discharge (Geerts *et al.* 2008).

Urological surgery

- Patients should be offered mechanical prophylaxis (NICE 2007). The ACCP (2008) recommend that patients undergoing transurethral or other low-risk urology procedures should avoid specific prophylaxis and aim for early and persistent mobilization.
- Patients with one or more risk factor for VTE should be offered LMWH (NICE 2007) or UFH combined with GCS (Geerts *et al.* 2008).

Laparoscopic surgery

- Routine thromboprophylaxis is not recommended in these patients – other than aggressive mobilization (Geerts *et al.* 2008).
- Those patients with additional VTE risk factors should receive one or more of the following: LMWH, UFH, GCS or IPC (Geerts *et al.* 2008).

Neurosurgery (including spinal surgery)

Patients having neurosurgery are known to be at moderately increased risk of postoperative VTE; however, given the risk of intracranial or spinal bleeding from the use of anticoagulation, mechanical prophylaxis is preferred (SIGN 2002).

- Patients undergoing spinal surgery with no additional risk factors should be encouraged to mobilize early, but routine use of thromboprophylaxis is not advised. Patients undergoing major neurosurgery, however, should use some form of thromboprophylaxis (Geerts *et al.* 2008).
- Patients having neurosurgery with one or more risk factors for VTE should be offered mechanical prophylaxis and LMWH (NICE 2007)
- Patients with ruptured cranial or spinal vascular malformations (e.g. brain aneurysms) should not be offered pharmacological prophylaxis until the lesion has been secured (NICE 2007). Mechanical prophylaxis can be used (Geerts *et al.* 2008).
- High-risk neurosurgical patients can be given UFH or postoperative LMWH (Geerts *et al.* 2008) but there is an increased risk of bleeding (SIGN 2002).

Medical patients

The United Kingdom National Venous Thromboembolism Registry recorded 2720 cases of VTE between December 2001 and November 2003; 323 (12%) of these cases had recently had a hospital stay as a medical inpatient [compared to the 265 (9.7%) who had undergone recent surgery], suggesting that acute medical illness is an independent risk factor for VTE (O'Shaughnessy *et al.* 2004). Prior to the publicity generated from the House of Commons Health Committee Report in 2005, the use of thromboprophylaxis in medical patients was not widely practised. Postulated reasons for this were lack of evidence for thromboprophylaxis in medical patients, combined with a greater heterogeneity of medical patients compared with surgical patients, which was thought to make risk assessment difficult (Leizorovicz *et al.* 2004b).

It is now well recognized that hospitalized medical patients are at an increased risk of thrombosis, and that implementing thromboprophylaxis in this group can significantly reduce the burden of disease due to VTE (Geerts *et al.* 2008).

Current recommendations from the ACCP

- Prophylaxis with UFH or LMWH should be given to acutely ill medical patients admitted to hospital with congestive heart failure or severe respiratory disease, or patients confined to bed and having one or more additional risk factor (including active cancer, previous VTE, sepsis, acute neurological disease or inflammatory bowel disease).
- Mechanical prophylaxis can be used in patients in whom there is a contraindication to anticoagulation (Geerts *et al.* 2008).

There are groups of medical patients who are at permanent risk for VTE who, it could be argued, should be on long-term thromboprophylaxis, such as patients with limited mobility who live in nursing homes, or need hospitalization for chronic conditions such as paraplegia. There are currently no guidelines in place for such patients, since no studies have been carried out to assess the benefit of long-term prophylaxis (Leizorovicz *et al.* 2004b). This is an area where further research is needed.

Malignancy

Cancer patients have a significantly increased risk of VTE (Heit *et al.* 2000) and patients with cancer undergoing surgery, receiving chemotherapy or with a central venous line *in situ* are at even greater risk (Geerts *et al.* 2008). Current guidelines from the ACCP for patients with malignancy include:

- Cancer patients undergoing surgery receive prophylaxis that is appropriate for their current risk state (see the guidelines above in each of the surgical specialties).

- Hospitalized cancer patients bedridden with an acute medical illness should receive prophylaxis that is appropriate for their current risk state (see the guidelines above in medical patients).
- Prophylaxis should not be routinely used to prevent VTE related to indwelling central venous catheters in cancer patients and the used of fixed-dose warfarin for this indication should also be avoided (Geerts et al. 2008)

Critical care

Patients admitted to an intensive care unit often have multiple risk factors for VTE and current guidance from the ACCP advises that a VTE risk assessment is carried out on admission.

- Those patients at high risk of bleeding should receive mechanical prophylaxis until the bleeding risk decreases.
- Patients at a moderate risk of VTE (such as postoperative or medically ill patients) should receive either UFH or LMWH prophylaxis.
- Higher risk patients (such as following major trauma or orthopaedic surgery) should receive LMWH prophylaxis.

Stroke

The optimal form of pharmacological prophylaxis in stroke patients remains unknown, since even low-dose heparin is associated with a significant number of symptomatic intracranial and extracranial bleeds (IST 1997). Early treatment with aspirin is advocated, once intracranial haemorrhage is excluded, to prevent further cardiovascular events. The use of prophylactic LMWH compared to UFH in ischaemic stroke has been associated with a reduction in VTE, with no demonstrable increased incidence of bleeding in some studies (Shorr et al. 2008). However, national guidelines recommend against the routine use of heparin in acute stroke in view of bleeding risk. In those patients judged to be at higher than average risk of VTE and lower than average risk of haemorrhagic complications, LMWH can be considered (SIGN 2002).

Graduated compression stockings and intermittent pneumatic compression devices have proven efficacy in peri-operative patients (Wells et al. 1994), but there is a paucity of evidence for their benefits in stroke patients (Muir et al. 2000). The recent CLOTS 1 trial, the first large assessment of the safety and efficacy of GCS in patients with recent stroke, suggest that GCS do not work and are associated with a four fold increase in skin ulcers and necrosis and they may promote lower limb ischaemia (Bath PMW et al. 2009). Previous guidelines have suggested that GCS may provide some benefit in stroke patients (SIGN 1999, Geerts *et al.* 2008), and it is now being suggested that these guidelines should be updated. Early mobilization and hydration should be encouraged as practicable to further reduce the risk of thrombosis (Indredavik *et al.* 1999).

Pregnancy and the puerperium

A positive history of VTE should be elicited from women on their first antenatal visit and all women with a personal history or family history of VTE should be offered screening for thrombophilias. Regular assessment of VTE risks factors should continue throughout pregnancy (SIGN 2002).

In patients with previous VTE, management needs to be individualized (see Table 3.2, p. 50). In patients whose previous VTE was attributed to temporary risk factors that are no longer present, LMWH prophylaxis is not routinely recommended but GCS should be considered (SIGN 2002).

Women with idiopathic VTE should start LMWH prophylaxis as early as possible in pregnancy, combined with GCS. LMWH is preferred to UFH, as there is more safety data available (SIGN 2002; RCOG 2004). Patients with a known thrombophilic defect and/or on long-term anticoagulant drugs should be managed by an experienced unit.

Prior to delivery, women who have requested epidural anaesthesia should stop anticoagulation when labour starts – spinal anaesthesia should not be given for 10–12 hours following LMWH administration (SIGN 2002). All women with a prior history of VTE should receive thromboprophylaxis post partum, as should women with known thrombophilia and other thrombotic risk factors. The first dose of LMWH should be given 3–6 hours after delivery and continued until discharge from hospital (SIGN 2002). Anticoagulation is recommended for a minimum of 6 weeks in patients with previous VTE or thrombophilia. Warfarin should be avoided during pregnancy but is safe after delivery and during breastfeeding (RCOG 2004).

Trauma and spinal cord injury

VTE is a common complication of major trauma (Geerts *et al.* 1994); however, due to the nature of injuries sustained by trauma patients, there are often contraindications to the use of anticoagulation, such as spinal, abdominal or intracranial injuries. Prophylaxis following trauma was first recommended 60 years ago (Bauer 1944); however, there are very few randomized trials in this particular group. Mechanical prophylaxis is widely used to avoid bleeding risks. The ACCP advocates this and, in the absence of any major contraindications, recommends LMWH prophylaxis in trauma patients (including burns patients) with at least one risk factor for VTE (Geerts *et al.* 2008).

Patients with spinal cord injury are at particular risk of VTE, and thromboprophylaxis with LMWH rather than UFH is advised. GCS can be used where anticoagulants are contraindicated (Geerts *et al.* 2008).

During the rehabilitation phase following acute spinal cord injury or trauma, continuation of LMWH prophylaxis or conversion to an oral VKA (target INR 2.5) is advised (Geerts *et al.* 2008).

Long-distance travel

For long-distance travellers on flights of more than 6 hours duration, passengers should avoid constrictive clothing around the lower extremities, ensure that they are well hydrated and participate in frequent calf muscle stretching. In those travellers with additional risk factors for VTE, if active prophylaxis is considered, then it should be in the form of properly fitted GCS or a single prophylactic dose of LMWH prior to departure. The use of aspirin is not advised by the ACCP (Geerts *et al.* 2008) but is advocated by SIGN (2002). See Chapter 3 for further information.

Case study 1: thromboprophylaxis in practice

Throughout the course of your day, you come into contact with the following patients.

Which patients do you think should be started on LMWH thromboprophylaxis?

(a) A 63 year-old woman with breast cancer, admitted for a course of chemotherapy.
(b) A 32 year-old man awaiting knee arthroplasty.
(c) A 96 year-old man who is medically well, admitted for 'social reasons' (awaiting placement in a nursing home for advanced Alzheimer's disease).
(d) A 40 year-old woman with cellulitis, diagnosed with DVT a month ago and on warfarin.
(e) A 51 year-old woman with pneumonia and known congestive heart failure.

All the patients should be subject to an individual risk assessment with analysis of their VTE risk factors balanced by their bleeding risk.

(a) This patient is hospitalized, over 60 years old, has cancer and is about to undergo chemotherapy, so, regardless of her other risk factors, she is already a candidate for pharmacological prophylaxis.

(b) This patient is young but is in hospital for orthopaedic surgery, which immediately puts him at high risk of developing DVT.

(c) An elderly patient with no acute medical illness but with Alzheimer's disease would not be someone who should be automatically commenced on LMWH unless VTE risk factors emerge during a comprehensive risk assessment. This patient is at risk of falls, since he is likely to remain mobile, which puts him at increased risk of bleeding on LMWH therapy.

(d) This lady with cellulitis is in hospital with an acute medical illness, but she is already being anticoagulated with warfarin, so as long as she is continuing to take this and her INR is within range, there is no need to put her on LMWH as well.

(e) This lady is hospitalized with an acute medical illness and already has heart failure, which puts her at an increased risk for VTE. LMWH should be considered in her case.

Patients who have contraindications to pharmocological methods should be issued with mechanical prophylaxis (ensuring they have no contraindications to this) and advised to ambulate as much as possible, or to engage in leg exercises if immobility is an issue. Patients should also remain adequately hydrated.

Conclusion

Prevention is always better than cure – this is espcially true when dealing with VTE. Thromboprophylaxis has been proved to be effective in reducing VTE episodes, contributing to a reduced mortality rate and a reduction in morbidity from PTS and recurrent VTE. Various methods of thromboprophylaxis are in use to suit the different needs and contraindications of different patient groups. VTE should be considered in all patients admitted to hospital and thromboprophylaxis initiated according to need.

References

Bath PMW, England TJ (2009) Effectiveness of thigh length graduated compression stockings to reduce the risk of deep vein thrombosis after stroke (CLOTS trial 1): a multicentre, randomised controlled trial. *Lancet* **373** (9679): 1958–1965.

Bauer G (1944) Thrombosis following leg injuries. *Acta Chirurgica Scandinavica* **90**: 229–248.

Blann AD, Lip GY (2006) Venous thromboembolism. *British Medical Journal* **332**: 215–219.

Bounameaux H, Perneger T (2002) Fondaparinux: a new synthetic pentasaccharide for thrombosis prevention. *Lancet* **359**: 1710–1711.

Canavarro K (1946) Early post-operative ambulation. *Annals of Surgery* **124**: 180–181.

Department of Health (DH) (2007) *Report of the Independent Expert Working Group on the Prevention of Venous Thromboembolism in Hospitalized Patients*. Department of Health, London. http://www.dh.gov.uk/en/Publicationsandstatistics/PublicationsPolicyAndGuidance/DH_073944

Fedullo PF, Auger WR, Kerr KM *et al.* (2001) Chronic thromboembolic pulmonary hypertension. *New England Journal of Medicine* **345**: 1465–1472.

Geerts WH, Code KI, Jay RM *et al.* (1994) A prospective study of venous thromboembolism after major trauma. *New England Journal of Medicine* **331**: 1601–1606.

Geerts WH, Bergqvist D, Pineo GF *et al.* (2008) Prevention of venous thromboembolism. American College of Chest Physicians: evidence based clinical practice guidelines, 8th Edition. *Chest* **133**: 381–453S.

Heit JA, Silverstein MD, Mohr DN *et al.* (1999) Predictors of survival after deep vein thrombosis and pulmonary embolism. A population-based cohort study. *Archives of Internal Medicine* **159**: 445–453.

Heit JA, Silverstein MD, Mohr DN *et al.* (2000) Risk factors for deep vein thrombosis and pulmonary embolism: a population based case control study. *Archives of Internal Medicine* **160**: 809–815.

Hopkins NF, Wolfe JH (1992) ABC of vascular diseases: deep venous insufficiency and occlusion. *British Medical Journal* **304**: 107–110.

House of Commons Health Committee (HCHC) (2005) *The Prevention of Venous Thromboembolism in Hospitalised Patients*. HC99. Stationery Office, London. Available at: www.publications.parliament.uk/pa/cm200405/cmselect/cmhealth/99/9902.htm*evidence_downloaded_29

Indredavik B, Bakke F, Slordahl SA *et al.* (1999) Treatment in a combined acute and rehabilitation stroke unit: which aspects are most important? *Stroke* **30**: 917–923.

International Stroke Trial Collaborative Group (IST) (1997) The International Stroke Trial. A randomised trial of aspirin, subcutaneous heparin, both or neither among 19,435 patients with acute ischemic stroke. *Lancet* **349**: 1569–1581.

Kahn SR, Ginsberg JF (2002a) The post-thrombotic syndrome: current knowledge, controversies and directions for future research. *Blood Review* **16**: 155–165.

Kahn SR, Hirsch A, Shrier I (2002b) Effect of post-thrombotic syndrome on health-related quality of life after deep vein thrombosis. *Archives of Internal Medicine* **162**: 1144–1148.

Kahn SR, Ginsberg JS (2004) Relationship between deep venous thrombosis and the postthrombotic syndrome. *Archives of Internal Medicine* **164**: 17–26.

Kahn SR, Desmarais S, Ducruet T *et al.* (2006) Comparison of the Villalta and Ginsberg clinical scales to diagnose the post-thrombotic syndrome: correlation with patient reported disease burden and venous valvular reflux. *Journal of Thrombosis and Haemostasis* **4**: 907–908.

Kearon C (2003) Natural history of venous thromboembolism. *Circulation* **107**: 22–30.

Leizorovicz A, Cohen AT, Turpie AGG *et al.* (2004a) Randomised, placebo-controlled trial of dalteparin for the prevention of venous thromboembolism in acutely ill medical patients. *Circulation* **110**: 874–879.

Leizorovicz A, Mismetti P (2004b) Preventing venous thromboembolism in medical patients. *Circulation* **110**(Suppl IV): 13–19.

Mismetti P, Laporte-Simitsidis S, Tardy B *et al.* (2000) Prevention of VTE in internal medicine with unfractionated or low molecular weight heparins: a meta-analysis of randomised clinical trials. *Thrombosis and Haemostasis* **83**: 14–19.

Mismetti P, Laporte-Simitsidis S, Zufferey P *et al.* (2004) Prevention of venous thromboembolism in orthopedic surgery with vitamin K antagonists: a meta analysis. *Journal of Thrombosis and Haemostasis* **2**: 1058–1070.

Anonymous (2002) Fondaparinux (Arixtra), a new anticoagulant. *Medical Letter on Drugs and Therapeutics* **44**: 43.

Muir KW, Watt A, Baxter G *et al.* (2000) Randomised trial of graded compression stockings for prevention of deep vein thrombosis after acute stroke. *Quarterly Journal of Medicine* **93**: 359–364.

National Institute for Health and Clinical Excellence (NICE) (2007) *Venous Thromboembolism (Deep Vein Thrombosis and Pulmonary Embolism) in Patients Undergoing Surgery.* NICE, London. Available at: http://guidance.nice.org.uk/CG046

O'Shaughnessy D, Rose P, Scriven N *et al.* (2004) Second Venous Thromboembolism Registry Report (VERITY). Dendrite Clinical Systems, Henley-on-Thames.

Pengo V, Lensing AW, Prins MH *et al.* (2004) Incidence of chronic thromboembolic pulmonary hypertension after pulmonary embolism. *New England Journal of Medicine* **350**: 2257–2264.

Pulmonary Embolism Prevention (PEP) trial (2000) Prevention of pulmonary embolism and deep vein thrombosis with low dose aspirin. *Lancet* **355**: 1295–1305.

Phillips T, Stanton B, Provan A *et al.* (1994) A study of the impact of leg ulcers on quality of life: financial, social and psychologic implications. *Journal of the American Academy of Dermatology* **31**: 49–53.

Prandoni P, Lensing AW, Cogo A *et al.* (1996) The long term clinical course of acute deep vein thrombosis. *Annals of Internal Medicine* **125**: 1–7.

Prandoni P, Lensing AW, Prins MH *et al.* (2004) Below knee elastic compression stockings to prevent the post thrombotic syndrome: a randomised, controlled trial. *Annals of Internal Medicine* **141**: 249–256.

Royal College of Obstetricians and Gynaecologists (RCOG) (2004) Thromboprophylaxis during pregnancy, labour and after vaginal delivery. Guideline No. 37. Available at: http://www.rcog.org.uk/files/rcog-corp/uploaded-files/GT37Thromboprophylaxis2004.pdf

Samama MM, Cohen AT, Darmon JY *et al.* (1999) A comparison of enoxaparin with placebo for the prevention of venous thromboembolism in acutely ill medical patients: Prophylaxis in Medical Patients with Enoxaparin Study Group. *New England Journal of Medicine* **341**: 793–800.

The Scottish Intercollegiate Guidelines Network (SIGN) (1999) *National Clinical Guidelines on Antithrombotic Therapy.* University of Dundee. Available from: http://www.sign.ac.uk/pdf/sign36.pdf

The Scottish Intercollegiate Guidelines Network (SIGN) (2002) National Clinical Guidelines on Prophylaxis of Venous Thromboembolism. University of Dundee. Available from: http://www.sign.ac.uk/pdf/sign62.pdf

Shorr AF, Jackson WL, Sherner JH *et al.* (2008) Differences between low molecular weight and unfractionated heparin for venous thromboembolism prevention following ischemic stroke. *Chest* **133**: 149–155.

Stein PD, Henry JW (1995) Prevalence of acute pulmonary embolism among patients in a general hospital and at autopsy. *Chest* **108**: 978–981.

Villalta S, Bagatella P, Piccioli A *et al.* (1994) Assessment of validity and reproducibility of a clinical scale for the post-thrombotic syndrome. *Haemostasis* **24**: 158a.

Wells PS, Lensing AWA, Hirsh J (1994) Graduated compression stockings in the prevention of postoperative venous thromboembolism: a meta analysis. *Archives of Internal Medicine* **154**: 67–72.

Wilkins RW, Stanton JR (1953) Elastic stockings in the prevention of pulmonary embolism. A progress report. *New England Journal of Medicine* **248**: 1087–1090.

Wright H (1956) Effects of post-operative bedrest and early ambulation on the rate of venous blood flow. *Lancet* **1**: 222.

Deep vein thrombosis

Overview

Deep vein thrombosis (DVT) usually begins when small deposits of fibrin collect in the deep veins of the extremities, as a result of slow blood flow, combined with local activation of the clotting cascade. DVT can be asymptomatic, but the classic symptoms of calf pain, swelling, increased skin temperature, superficial venous dilatation and (occasionally) pitting oedema usually occur when a thrombus becomes large enough to cause blood outflow problems (Gorman *et al.* 2000). Complete occlusion of a vein is rare, but can lead to a cyanotic discoloration of the limb accompanied by severe oedema.

Clinical diagnosis of DVT is unreliable, so a combination of diagnostic investigations is usually performed, the gold standard being contrast venography. Since this procedure is invasive and expensive, it is rarely used (Tovey *et al.* 2003). In current practice, an algorithm combining pre-test probability, D-dimer testing and ultrasonography has been found to be a safe and convenient method of excluding DVT (Scarvelis *et al.* 2006).

Anticoagulation is the mainstay of treatment and interventions such as thrombolysis and inferior vena cava filters are reserved

Venous Thromboembolism: A Nurses Guide to Prevention and Management   By Ellen Welch
© 2010 John Wiley & Sons, Ltd.

for special situations (Kearon *et al.* 2008). The use of low molecular weight heparin allows the majority of patients with DVT to be managed as outpatients (Van Dongen *et al.* 2004). The duration of oral anticoagulation therapy depends on the likely aetiology of the primary event, and further research is needed to determine the patients who are at an increased risk of recurrence, who would benefit from an extended duration of therapy.

This chapter explores the condition in further detail.

Signs and symptoms

Symptoms of deep vein thrombosis (DVT) tend to be dependent on the degree of obstruction to venous flow and vessel wall inflammation (Gorman *et al.* 2000) and the more proximal and occlusive the thrombus, the more marked are the symptoms and physical signs (Browse *et al.* 1988). Unfortunately clinical diagnosis is notoriously unreliable, since DVTs are often 'silent' (asymptomatic) and many non-thrombotic conditions can produce signs and symptoms suggestive of DVT. One study showed that 75% of outpatients who presented with signs and symptoms suggestive of DVT did not have the disease (Wells *et al.* 1995).

Classic symptoms (see Box 5.1) include pain, swelling and discoloration of the effected extremity (Figure 5.1 illustrates a left proximal DVT). Examination may reveal tenderness on compression of the calf muscles, or tenderness over the main vessels of the thigh.

Pitting oedema of the ankle is a significant indicator of thrombosis in 70% of cases, especially if it is unilateral, while oedema of the calf

---

Box 5.1 Clinical features of DVT

- Calf pain and/or tenderness.
- Swelling with pitting oedema.
- Swelling below the knee (distal DVT) and up to the groin (proximal DVT).
- Superficial venous dilatation.
- Increased skin temperature.
- Cyanosis/discoloration (with severe obstruction).

(Adapted from Gorman *et al.* 2000)

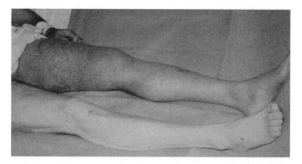

Figure 5.1 Left proximal DVT with calf swelling, pitting oedema and skin discoloration. Included with the permission of the King's Thrombosis Centre.

and foot may indicate that the thrombus has extended into the popliteal vein (McLachlin *et al.* 1962). Entire leg swelling is associated with iliofemoral or vena caval thrombosis.

If there is significant venous outflow obstruction, the skin may feel warm, with superficial venous dilatation, and the thrombosed vein may be palpable under the skin as a hard cord (Hirsh *et al.* 1986). The calf muscles may feel hard if there is extensive intramuscular thrombosis (Browse *et al.* 1988).

Pain occurring on dorsiflexion of the foot (Homan's sign) is notoriously unreliable and can occur with any of the conditions listed in Box 5.2 (Ramzi *et al.* 2004).

Skin discoloration may be observed in patients with DVT. A 'white leg' (phlegmasia alba dolens) is often seen on examination, thought to be caused by extensive oedema, which masks the capillary circulation of the skin, and is usually due to an iliofemoral thrombosis (Homans 1928). Phlegmasia cerulea dolens (blue, painful leg) is an uncommon manifestation of DVT resulting from massive thrombosis compromising venous drainage, causing ischaemia which can progress to gangrene if the outflow obstruction is not relieved (see Figure 5.2). Venous gangrene develops when the venous outflow is so severely reduced that the arterial inflow becomes obstructed. This results in the tips of the toes becoming blue, then black, and the skin may blister. All the toes are usually affected (unlike arterial gangrene) and may spread to affect the dorsal surface of the foot (Browse *et al.* 1988). It is often difficult to palpate foot pulses in a limb with venous gangrene or phlegmasia cerulea dolens. A low-grade fever is often found in patients with DVT and many patients who present with superficial thrombophlebitis often have concurrent asymptomatic DVT (Bergqvist *et al.* 1986; Feied 2005).

Box 5.2 Possible causes of pain or swelling of the lower limb

- Deep vein thrombosis.
- Superficial thrombophlebitis.
- Post-thrombotic syndrome.
- Chronic venous insufficiency.
- Venous obstruction.
- Cellulitis.
- Ruptured Baker's cyst.
- Torn gastrocnemius muscle.
- Fracture.
- Acute arthritis of the knee.
- Myositis ossificans.
- Rapidly growing sarcoma.
- Calf haematoma.
- Acute arterial ischaemia.
- Lymphoedema.
- Hypoproteinaemia (e.g. cirrhosis, nephrotic syndrome).

(Tovey *et al.* 2003) reproduced with permission from the BMJ group

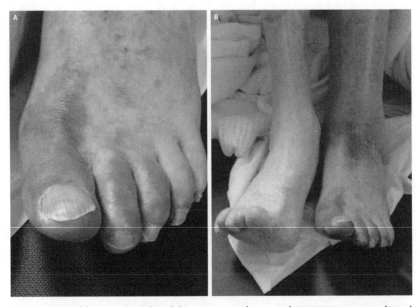

Figure 5.2 Phlegmasia cerulea dolens. From Barham *et al.* (2007) Images in clinical medicine: phlegmasia cerulea dolens. *New England Journal of Medicine* **356**(3): e3. Copyright © 2007, Massachusetts Medical Society. All rights reserved.

A thrombus involving the iliac bifurcation, the pelvic veins, or the vena cava may produce leg oedema that usually is bilateral rather than unilateral and may be mistaken for fluid overload characteristic of other disease processes. Severe venous congestion produces a clinical appearance that can be indistinguishable from the appearance of cellulitis. If diagnosis was not difficult enough already, patients with primary DVT often develop a secondary cellulitis, while patients with primary cellulitis often develop a secondary DVT (Bersier *et al.* 2003).

The proximal veins of the leg, namely the popliteal vein and the superficial femoral vein, are most commonly affected by DVT (see Figure 2.1, p. 22). An autopsy study looking for the source of fatal PEs showed that one-third of fatal emboli arose from the calf veins (Havig 1977). Studies since then, however, have shown that isolated DVTs in calf veins are thought to pose little risk of extension or pulmonary embolism in the short term. In symptomatic patients only 20% of thrombi detected by ultrasound are isolated to the calf and only 20–30% of these calf thrombi will eventually extend to the proximal veins (Scarvelis *et al.* 2006). Calf veins are smaller, with a slower blood flow and more anatomical variation than the proximal veins, which leads to technically inadequate studies with ultrasound. Many centres therefore limit ultrasound imaging to the proximal veins, where the sensitivity of the test is 97% compared with only 73% in the calf veins (Kearon *et al.* 1998a). In asymptomatic patients, the sensitivity of ultrasound is even lower, in the range 33–58% (ATS 1999).

Reliability of clinical signs

It is repeatedly reported that the clinical symptoms and signs associated with DVT are unreliable, and even in the presence of the 'classical' symptoms, in a high-risk patient it is difficult to definitively say 'This patient has a DVT' (Wheeler 1985). Several studies were carried out in the 1960s when imaging studies became more readily available, which allow us to consider certain signs and symptoms as being more reliable than others.

Flanc *et al.* (1968) evaluated symptoms in patients with DVT confirmed with both phlebography and the fibrogen uptake test and it was found that 25% had calf tenderness, 34% had a detectable difference in temperature of the affected limb; 52% had mild unilateral ankle oedema and 68% had some induration of the calf muscles. A similar study by Kakkar *et al.* (1970) showed that the presenting symptoms in his patients were calf tenderness in 66%, swelling in 10% and PE in another 10%. Calf swelling was found to be the most indicative sign of DVT in reports by McLachlin *et al.* (1962), with 80% of his proven DVT patients displaying swelling, while local tenderness was consistent with the diagnosis in only 50%.

Therefore, calf swelling and tenderness with associated ankle oedema can be considered the 'most reliable' signs of DVT, but their presence alone does not reliably confirm or exclude DVT but indicates the need for further evaluation (ATS 1999). Box 5.3 outlines a method for clinical examination of the lower limb. Due to this lack of clinical certainty, diagnosticians have developed clinical prediction tools that combine the results of carefully defined signs and symptoms to stratify patients into groups at risk of DVT (Wells PS *et al.* 1997, 1998). This avoids missing those patients in which DVT may be silent, and avoids costly, unnecessary tests on patients with swollen legs due to an entirely different aetiology. The most common alternative diagnoses are listed below.

Box 5.3 Simple examination of the lower limbs

For completeness, combine lower limb examination with a general examination, vital signs and full history. Always assess patients' gait as they walk in the room. Be systematic, compare both sides. Start by inspecting for discomfort, muscle wasting, swelling, discoloration, venous dilatation, varicose veins or deformity. Move on to palpation. Start by measuring the circumference of both calves by placing a tape measure 6 inches (15 cm) below the centre of the patella (Swarczinski *et al.* 1991). Assess the soft tissue for warmth, erythema and oedema and palpate for calf tenderness or palpable veins. Test the range of movement of the limb. Pulses should be palpated and a neurological assessment made.

Antiquated clinical tests

Homan's sign, also known as the dorsiflexion sign, is a method of testing for calf tenderness that was disowned by its creator as being unreliable. The test involves passively dorsi-flexing the foot of a supine patient (moving the patient's foot towards his/her head). A positive test will elicit pain in the soleus and gastrocnemius muscles. Previously this was thought to be indicative of the presence of venous thrombosis, but any conditions causing irritability of the posterior muscles can be 'Homans-positive' (Ramzi *et al.* 2004). In the prospective studies of deep vein thrombosis, diagnosed with imaging techniques, the overall finding is that physical examination has both low sensitivity and low specificity (Sandler *et al.* 1984; O'Donnell *et al.* 1980; Mclachlin *et al.* 1962). The Loewenberg test was

---

created as an attempt to quantify Homans' sign and involved eliciting tenderness by inflating a pneumatic tourniquet around the calf muscles and inflating it to determine at which pressure pain occurred – this test has also been proved to be unreliable (Makin 1968).

If thoracic outlet syndrome is suspected in patients with upper extremity DVT, the hand and arm should be inspected for evidence of atrophy and the supraclavicular fossa should be palpated for brachial plexus discomfort. There are two provocative tests that can be carried out to elicit symptoms of thoracic outlet obstruction. To perform Adson's test, the examiner extends the patient's arm on the affected side while asking the patient to extend the neck and rotate the head towards the same side. Compression of the subclavian artery is suggested by weakening of the radial pulse on deep inspiration while in this position. Wright's manoeuvre tests for reproducibility of symptoms and weakening of the radial pulse with abduction of the patient's shoulder, with the humerus held in external rotation (Parziale *et al.* 2000).

Differential diagnosis

Superficial thrombophlebitis (Figure 5.3)

Superficial thrombophlebitis, like DVT, is caused by the presence of a blood clot in a vein, occluding the flow of blood. It tends to affect the visible veins just under the skin. Typically the area of inflammation is

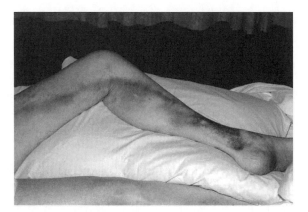

Figure 5.3 Superficial thrombophlebitis. From Lucia *et al.* (2001) Images in clinical medicine: superficial thrombophlebitis. *New England Journal of Medicine* **344**(16): 1214. Copyright © 2001, Massachusetts Medical Society. All rights reserved.

erythematous, tender and warm to the touch, and examination reveals a palpable 'cord-like' thrombosed vein. Thrombophlebitis of the leg is often associated with pre-existing varicosities and manifests when combined with trauma or immobilization, while upper limb thrombophlebitis is often iatrogenic, following an injection or an infusion. Treatment focuses on mobilization and compression accompanied by analgesia. Extensive thrombophlebitis may require heparinization and intercurrent infection requires early antibiotics (Diehm *et al.* 2000). A patient with superficial thrombophlebitis may also have a DVT. In a study of 562 patients with thrombophlebitis, 3.5% had a DVT in the same limb and 2.1% in the contralateral limb (Belcaro *et al.* 1999). In the past the term 'thrombophlebitis' was used to encompass DVT. The term is now reserved for thrombosis and phlebitis of the superficial veins, while 'DVT' is used to describe thrombosis of the deep veins (Browse *et al.* 1988).

Chronic venous insufficiency

Chronic venous insufficiency (CVI) was previously called post-thrombotic or post-phlebitic syndrome, since both terms referred to the aetiology of most cases. It is now recognized that not all cases of CVI are caused by VTE and some may be due to a congenital absence of venous valves. Chronic venous insufficiency can therefore be described as impaired venous return, sometimes causing lower extremity discomfort, oedema and skin changes. Post-thrombotic syndrome (PTS) is symptomatic chronic venous insufficiency after DVT. This condition is discussed further in Chapter 4.

Venous obstruction

Tumours in the pelvis or abdomen can cause obstruction to venous return, resulting in a backlog of fluid in the lower limbs. Patients with cancer are also prone to VTE, so distinguishing the aetiology of the swelling can be a challenge. Treatment that reduces the size of the obstructing mass will provide symptom relief.

Ruptured Baker's cyst

A Baker cyst is a reactive outpouching of the knee joint capsule and its presence implies chronic knee pathology, often arthritic in nature. The cyst is usually painless, but if it ruptures the leg swells and the pain is diffuse. This condition is difficult to distinguish from DVT, since is also presents with acute onset of pain and swelling in the calf, and only a few patients describe a history of previous arthritis in the knee (Simpson *et al.* 1980). Once rupture of the cyst has occurred there may be few physical signs of arthritis on examination of the joint, with no residual effusion or palpable cyst. Occasionally there will be bruising in the lower leg, anterior to the Achilles' tendon, but this often occurs days after the initial presentation (McFarlane *et al.* 1980). DVT may occur at the same time as a ruptured Baker's cyst, making the diagnosis even more difficult. To reach a diagnosis, arthography, ultrasound and phlebography may be required (Belch *et al.* 1981).

Torn gastrocnemius muscle

Usually presents with sudden-onset calf pain followed by swelling of the leg. The onset of the pain is usually more rapid than that of DVT and is associated with exercise. The plantaris tendon, which originates in the popliteal region, may also rupture due to sporting injury, resulting in a similar swelling and tenderness. Achilles tendon rupture may also present similarly, but can be distinguished by the patient's inability to plantar flex the foot, accompanied by a more distal and palpable defect of the tendon.

Fracture

A history of trauma is usually reported in patients with fractures. This is not always the case, however, in patients presenting with pathological fractures. Such patients often present with sudden-onset severe limb pain and swelling and fracture should be suspected in patients who have had previous treatment for malignancy. Radiographs of the limbs will confirm fracture, and it may be necessary to perform a radioactive isotope bone scan to search for evidence of other bony metastases.

Haematoma

A sudden acute bleed into soft tissues or into a joint, without a history of trauma, may occur in patients on anticoagulants or in those patients with coagulation disorders. The condition can be diagnosed by identification of a localized swelling combined with abnormal coagulation tests and a suspicious history. Computed tomography (CT) may occasionally be required to confirm diagnosis.

Acute arterial ischaemia

This condition commonly presents with the memorable collection of Ps – severe pain, pallor, pulselessness, paraesthesiae, paralysis and 'perishing' cold. Peripheral vascular disease is primarily due to atherosclerosis, a build-up of fatty deposits on the walls of the peripheral arteries. Acute ischaemia occurs with complete occlusion of the artery, which usually occurs secondary to emboli and requires prompt treatment to recanalize the vessel. Arterial occlusion and DVT can occasionally occur together but usually the presence of a pale, cold, pulseless limb indicates the correct diagnosis (Belch *et al.* 1981).

Lymphoedema and cellulitis

Lymphoedema is a condition in which the interstitial fluid of the body is unable to drain correctly, due to a compromised lymphatic system, and results in a swollen oedematous limb. The condition is mainly seen after lymph node dissection or radiation therapy for cancer but can be associated with any condition that causes damage to the lymphatic system. Patients with lymphoedema are prone to developing cellulitis, which causes pain, swelling and erythema (redness), which can be difficult to distinguish from DVT. Cellulitis (Figure 5.4) can also occur in patients who do not have lymphoedema and is usually identified by a spreading area of erythema, a high fever and raised inflammatory markers. Cellulitis literally means inflammation of the cells and is an infection of the dermis and subcutaneous tissues, usually caused by invasion of Gram-positive bacteria through broken skin. Red streaking

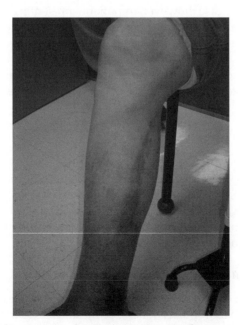

Figure 5.4 Cellulitis. Courtesy of Richard P. Usatine MD, from: www.dermatlas.net

in the skin proximal to the area of cellulitis is indicative of ascending lymphangitis, in which the infection is carried through the lymphatic system. The condition usually responds to a course of antibiotics.

Generalized oedema

A variety of conditions can lead to swelling of the legs which can be mistaken for DVT. Patients with congestive cardiac failure, renal failure and hypoproteinaemia (due to cirrhosis or nephrotic syndrome) tend to develop a bilateral, non-tender swelling of the legs. There is often a high incidence of VTE in patients with medical conditions that cause generalized oedema, and since DVTs can often be bilateral and painless, further investigations are often necessary to exclude the presence of a clot.

Arthritis

Pain from the knee joint can be referred to the calf, so an episode of acute arthritis may occasionally be mistaken for DVT. Usually the diagnosis can be made clinically by identifying the involvement of other joints, but even rheumatoid arthritis can sometimes be mono-articular, and misleading. Arthritic pain is usually worse on movement of the affected joint and with radiography and serological tests a diagnosis can usually be reached. Fibrinogen uptake tests performed on arthritic patients are a common cause of false-positive readings and a more definitive test is recommended (Poulose *et al.* 1976).

Investigations

The approach to diagnosing DVT has evolved over the last 10 years. Prior to 1995 the approach was to image all patients with suspected DVT and repeat imaging 1 week later if the results were negative (Wells *et al.* 2000). This method, however, was inefficient, since only 10–25% of patients with clinically suspected DVT were found to have the disorder and repeated testing was usually negative (Cogo *et al.* 1998; Wells *et al.* 1997).

The gold standard for establishing a diagnosis of DVT is contrast venography, but since this procedure is invasive, expensive and requires contrast media, it is inappropriate as an initial diagnostic test and is rarely used except when a definitive answer is required (Blann *et al.* 2006; Tovey *et al.* 2003). The accuracy of non-invasive tests varies according to whether the patient is symptomatic or asymptomatic, and with the type of DVT being diagnosed (i.e. proximal versus distal)

(Kearon *et al.* 1998a, 1998b). Compression ultrasonography is the chosen diagnostic test and relies on the lack of compressibility of a venous segment to confirm the presence of a DVT (Scarvelis *et al.* 2006). Ultrasonography is usually limited to the proximal veins of the leg for the reasons mentioned earlier. Where the distal calf has not been scanned, it has been established that serial testing should be undertaken by way of a repeat ultrasound scan 1 week later to detect DVT extending into the proximal veins (Cogo *et al.* 1998). Serial testing is only indicated in high-risk patients, since routine serial testing has been shown to be inefficient and inconvenient, with only 1–2% of patients with an initial negative ultrasound confirmed to have a proximal DVT on repeat testing (Wells *et al.* 1995; Kearon *et al.* 1998).

Clinical prediction rules

In view of the lack of reliable clinical signs and symptoms of DVT, it is good practice to use clinical prediction rules to establish a diagnosis of DVT. Patients can be categorized as having low, moderate or high probability of DVT, depending on their combination of signs, symptoms and risk factors and, depending on the category allocated to them, patients can then go on to have the appropriate investigations. It has been shown that patients with a low pretest probability can have DVT safely excluded on the basis of a single negative ultrasound result, thus saving time and money on unnecessary serial ultrasound testing (Wells *et al.* 1997). Multiple studies have proved that this model is effective (Scarvelis *et al.* 2006).

The most widely implemented scoring system in use in the United Kingdom is the Wells criteria (Table 5.1). Many NHS trusts have their own protocols in place, based on such scoring systems, to facilitate the diagnosis of DVT for junior doctors and to ensure they are managed appropriately. The Leeds Teaching Hospitals NHS Trust has developed such protocols for patients with suspected DVT presenting to the Emergency Department (ED), which allows selected patients (those with no comorbidities which require admission for more than 24 hours and patients not already using long-term warfarin) to be investigated and managed without the need for prolonged hospital admissions. At Leeds the Well's criteria are used combined with a proforma reminding physicians to enquire about other risk factors, such as oral contraceptives and pregnancy. Their management algorithm is outlined in Figure 5.5).

Clinical decisions units within the ED are wards which cater for various categories of patients, who can be discharged within 24–48 hours. The units have been used effectively in the United Kingdom to

Table 5.1 Wells' criteria

Clinical characteristics	Score
Active cancer (treatment ongoing, administered within previous 6 months or palliative)	1
Paralysis, paresis or recent plaster immobilization of lower extremity	1
Recently bedridden > 3 days or surgery within previous 12 weeks requiring general or regional anaesthesia	1
Localized tenderness along distribution of the deep venous system	1
Swelling of entire leg	1
Calf swelling >3 cm larger than asymptomatic side (measured 10 cm below tibial tuberosity)	1
Pitting oedema confined to the symptomatic leg	1
Collateral superficial veins (non-varicose)	1
Previous documented DVT	1
Alternative diagnosis at least as likely as DVT	−2

Key: score of 2 or more, DVT 'likely'; score of 2 or less, DVT 'unlikely'; OR clinical probability of DVT with score: 3+, high; 1–2, moderate; <1, low.
(Scarvelis *et al.* 2006) 'Copyright Canadian Medical Association Journal (Scarvelis and Wells 2006). This work is protected by copyright and the making of this copy was with the permission of Access Copyright. Any alteration of its content or further copying in any form whatsoever is strictly prohibited unless otherwise permitted by law.'

minimize clinical risk and prevent unnecessary prolonged hospital admissions (Hassan 2000). Such units are useful for patients with possible VTE, where there is often diagnostic uncertainty. Low-risk patients may have been discharged from ED in the past, resulting in significant complications for the patient if a PE is missed, along with damaging litigation for the health care providers involved (Ross *et al.* 2001). Use of VTE protocols within a clinical decisions unit minimizes this risk and allows patients to be rapidly investigated and appropriately managed.

What the investigations involve

Contrast venography
Venography (also called phlebography) remains the gold standard for the diagnosis of DVT, but is rarely used due to the accuracy of other non-invasive investigations. Performed by a competent technician, it is considered nearly 100% sensitive and specific, using the technique described by Rabinov and Paulin in the 1970s. The technique involves injection of a radio-opaque iodine-based contrast dye, generally into a superficial foot vein. X-ray images are then taken as the contrast is

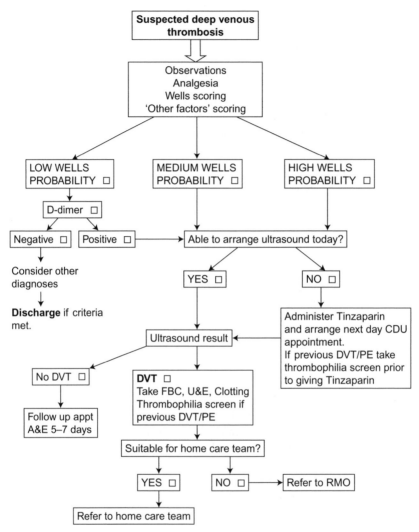

Figure 5.5 Management algorithm for suspected DVT. *RMO, resident medical officer. Reproduced with permission from the Leeds Teaching Hospitals Trust.

being injected. Adequate venography requires visualization of the deep venous system from the calf to the pelvic veins and inferior vena cava. A DVT can be reliably diagnosed if a constant intraluminal filling defect is present in two or more views (Rabinov *et al.* 1972). An abrupt cut off of a deep vein can also indicate the presence of a thrombus, but requires cautious interpretation in patients with previous DVT (ATS 1999). A limitations of venography is its invasiveness, which may result

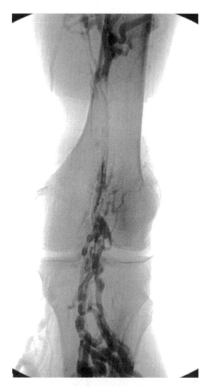

Figure 5.6 Venogram showing a popliteal DVT. From Tovey *et al.* (2003) *British Medical Journal* **326**: 1180–1184. Reproduced with permission from the BMJ Publishing Group.

in pain, phlebitis or hypersensitivity reactions. Occasionally, DVT may result from performing the procedure itself, and toxicity of the contrast agent may result in nephrotoxicity or cardiotoxicity. Such adverse effects mean that the procedure is relatively contraindicated in patients with chronic renal insufficiency. Allergic reactions can be minimized using antihistamines and corticosteroids. Venography is widely available, although it is more expensive than impedance plethysmography or ultrasonography, and remains the most sensitive test for calf DVT (ATS 1999) (Figure 5.6).

Plethysmography
Plethysmography (or phlebography) describes the process of recording change in the size of the limb due to tissue fluid or pooled blood in the veins. It is a non-invasive alternative to venography, requiring less technical training to perform, and is portable and less expensive but not as accurate at detecting small or non-occlusive thrombi (Browse

et al. 1988). There are several ways of performing this measurement. Impedance plethysmography measures the rate of venous return from the lower limbs, relying on the principle that the volume of blood in the leg affects its ability to conduct an electrical current. A cuff is inflated around the thigh to obstruct venous outflow, two electrodes are placed along the calf and an electrical current is applied and monitored. As blood accumulates in the calf below the inflated cuff, impedance (resistance of electrical current) between the calf and the electrodes falls. The sudden release of cuff pressure results in a sudden surge of blood flow proximally, resulting in a rapid increase in impedance. If DVT is present in a major vein draining the lower extremity, the rate of venous emptying (and the increase in impedance) is significantly slower. This technique will not detect thrombi that do not decrease the rate of venous outflow, such as calf thrombi, and there are multiple conditions that can result in false-positive results, such as obesity and pregnancy. The technique is useful in diagnosing recurrent DVT, since the initial positive findings revert to normal as the DVT resolves, and collateral circulation develops (ATS 1999).

Other methods of plethysmography available, but not as widely studied as impedance plethysmography, include digital photoplethysmography, which uses similar methods, basing the recording of venous filling upon the absorption of light by haemoglobin in the red cells, and computerized strain gauge plethysmography, which uses digital software to calculate blood flow measurements in the leg (Tovey *et al.* 2003).

Compression ultrasonography with venous imaging

Ultrasound is the most widely used imaging modality for the detection of DVT, due to its wide availability and its proven accuracy at diagnosing acute, symptomatic proximal DVT. It enables the examiner to identify other pathology that may be present, such as Baker's cysts, abscesses or haematoma (ATS 1999). Three techniques are in use.

Compression ultrasound is the simplest method of diagnosing thrombosis, by checking for non-compressibility of the vein. If no residual lumen is observed with a gentle probe pressure applied, then the vein is considered fully compressible, indicating that there is no occluding thrombus present (Figure 5.7).

Duplex ultrasound combines the two methods of Doppler venous flow detection with real-time sonography, providing additional information regarding blood flow. In normal veins, blood flow is spontaneous and phasic with respiration. When this pattern is lost, flow is continuous, indicative of venous outflow obstruction (Tovey *et al.* 2003).

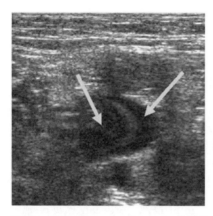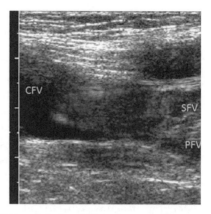

Figure 5.7 Ultrasound diagnosis of DVT. SFV occluded, with thrombus extending into CFV. Flow from PFV and SFV around thrombus. Included with the permission of the King's Thrombosis Centre.

The use of colour duplex imaging is identical to duplex ultrasound, but uses colour instead of a greyscale image, making identification of the vessels easier. Colour Doppler also aids diagnosis of non-occlusive thrombi. Simply put, the technique of ultrasonography involves tracing the path of the veins using an ultrasound transducer to compress the vessels, while Doppler studies confirm the presence of spontaneous venous flow.

Compression of the veins may be difficult in patients with tenderness, oedema or excess body fat, and in these situations, colour flow imaging will generally reveal venous filling. False-positive results may also be caused by compression of a vein by other pathology, such as a pelvic mass (Borgstede *et al.* 1992). False-negative studies have been reported in those patients with asymptomatic proximal DVT in the presence of calf DVT.

Ultrasound is considered unreliable in detecting iliac vein DVT and magnetic resonance imaging (MRI) or venography is recommended as an alternative (ATS 1999). Ultrasound also has its limitations when diagnosing recurrent DVT. Studies have revealed that up to 50% of patients with DVT diagnosed using ultrasound will have persistent sonographic changes (such as incomplete compressibility) at 6–12 months follow-up (Murphy *et al.* 1990; Heijboer *et al.* 1992). After several weeks, thrombi become adherent to the vessel wall and are less likely to embolize. When patients then present with recurrent symptoms, some will have new DVT, others will have postphlebitic syndrome. Ultrasound should not be considered reliable for the diagnosis of recurrent DVT unless the test has been shown to normalize prior to the suspected recurrence (ATS 1999).

Magnetic resonance imaging (MRI)

MRI provides detailed images of the body in any plane, producing excellent contrast between the different soft tissues of the body. It uses a magnetic field to make all the hydrogen protons in the body align to the direction of the field. A second radiofrequency electromagnetic field is applied, causing the protons to absorb some of its energy. When the field is turned off, the protons release this energy, which is then detected by the scanner, allowing an image of the body to be made up. MRI has been found to be at least 90% sensitive and specific for the detection of acute, symptomatic proximal DVT (Erdman *et al.* 1990). Information regarding its role as a screening test is asymptomatic patients is scarce (ATS 1999). It does not rely on compression; it avoids the use of ionizing radiation or contrast and is useful if an alternative diagnosis is suspected. It can visualize difficult areas, such as the upper extremities or the pelvic vessels, and has a role to play in distinguishing between acute and chronic DVT. There are contraindications to the procedure, however, such as claustrophobia, massive obesity and the inability to cooperate. Particular care is needed to determine those patients who have implanted metallic devices from previous injuries or surgeries. MRI is not always readily available and has the disadvantage of being an expensive procedure to perform (ATS 1999).

What is D-dimer testing?

D-dimer is a product of the breakdown of a cross-linked fibrin blood clot, produced when fibrin is degraded by plasmin. Levels of D-dimer are typically elevated in patients with acute VTE, but are also elevated in a number of other non-thrombotic conditions, such as after major surgery or recent trauma and haemorrhage, during pregnancy and in patients with cancer (Kelly *et al.* 2002b). The factors affecting raised D-dimer levels are outlined in Box 5.4. D-dimer assays are generally very sensitive but very non-specific markers of VTE and are valuable as a 'rule-out' test, since they have a high negative predictive value. If combined with appropriate pretest probability scoring and appropriate imaging, a negative D-dimer test can provide reassurance that VTE is unlikely. A positive test is not as useful, since there are many other possible causes for an elevation (Tovey *et al.* 2003).

Several D-dimer assays are in clinical use, the most common being laboratory-based enzyme-linked immunosorbent assay (ELISA) or a latex agglutination test. The VIDAS ELISA assay is the most exten-

---

Box 5.4 Factors affecting raised D-dimer levels

Levels are raised in many systemic illnesses associated with fibrin formation and subsequent breakdown, such as patients with severe infection, trauma or inflammatory disorders. In addition to VTE, D-dimer levels are raised in patients with:

- Disseminated intravascular coagulation (DIC).
- Vaso-occlusive sickle-cell crisis.
- Acute cerebrovascular accident.
- Acute myocardial infarction.
- Unstable angina.
- Pneumonia.
- Vasculitis.
- Superficial phlebitis.
- Many cancers, including lung, prostate, cervical and colorectal.

Other factors affecting D-dimer levels:

- The larger the clot, the higher the D-dimer level.
- Circulating D-dimer levels increase with age, pregnancy and smoking.
- D-dimer levels may not increase in an patient with acute VTE if they have impaired fibrinolytic activity.
- Levels decrease on heparin therapy and may reduce by two thirds in patients taking oral anticoagulants.
- The interval between onset of acute VTE and sample collection can affect the result.
- D-dimer levels may normalize in VTE of more than seven days duration.

(Sadosty *et al.* 2001) reproduced with permission from Elsevier

---

sively studied ELISA, providing a quantitative (numerical) result and displaying a greater sensitivity than the agglutination tests, which have the greatest specificity and provide a qualitative result (positive or negative) within 5 minutes (Kelly *et al.* 2002a). D-dimer concentration measured by ELISA has a 95% negative predictive power (Bounameaux *et al.* 1994). One study even suggested that PE can be safely excluded on the basis of a negative VIDAS test alone (Perrier *et al.* 1999), but caution is advised with this approach until further data is available. The SimpliRED test is less sensitive than the ELISA assays but appears safe in excluding VTE in those patients with a low pretest probability. Remember, these assays cannot be used in isolation, since VTE has occurred in up to 20% of patients with a high pretest probability but a negative SimpliRED D-dimer test (Kearon *et al.* 2001). Combination of a D-dimer with a formally derived pretest probability, however, can safely exclude the disease without the need for further imaging (Wells *et al.* 1998).

Bedside D-dimer assays such as the SimpliRED (agglutination test) and the Simplify (immunochromatography test) have been evaluated as a rapid screening test for DVT, and preliminary studies suggest they may be useful for emergency department diagnosis as part of a diagnostic algorithm, but further larger-scale studies are needed (Neale *et al.* 2004). ELISA assays differ between institutions and clinicians should know the diagnostic performance of the test used in their own workplace (Kelly *et al.* 2002).

There is some evidence to suggest that normal D-dimer levels measured after patients with DVT have finished their period of treatment with anticoagulation have a high negative predictive value for recurrent VTE (Palareti *et al.* 2002). Recent studies have shown that in patients who have completed three months of anticoagulation for a first episode unprovoked VTE, after two years of follow up a negative D-dimer result was associated with a 3.5% annual risk for recurrent disease, compared to an 8.9% annual risk in those with a positive D-dimer test (Verhovsek *et al.* 2008). It has been suggested that patients with an abnormal D-dimer one month after discontinuation of anticoagulation can reduce their risk of re-thrombosis by resuming anticoagulation (Palareti *et al.* 2006).

Treatment

The primary objective in the treatment of DVT is prevention of PE with anticoagulation to prevent clot extension. Methods of anticoagulation are therefore discussed in more detail in Chapter 7. Reducing morbidity and prevention of the postphlebitic syndrome are also major treatment aims and the latest summary of treatment recommendations compiled by the American College of Chest Physicians is outlined below.

Anticoagulation

Patients with acute DVT should be started on a vitamin K antagonist (VKA), together with short-term subcutaneous low molecular weight heparin (LMWH), unfractionated heparin (UH) or fondaparinux for five days until the INR is ≥2.0 for 24 hours (Kearon *et al.* 2008). Duration of therapy is three months for the first idiopathic episode and at least 6 months for other risk factors. The risk of bleeding should be balanced against the risk of further VTE and outpatient therapy is an option for stable patients (Kearon *et al.* 2008). Anticoagulation for patients with VTE is outlined in Chapter 7 in greater detail.

Catheter-directed thrombolysis (CDT) for acute DVT

Thrombolytic therapy has been found to be more effective than heparin at achieving vein patency; however, most patients with DVT have contraindications to its use and the longer the thrombus has been present, the less effective thrombolysis becomes. Venous thrombi in the legs are often large and associated with complete occlusion, meaning that the thrombolytic agent used may be unable to fully penetrate the entire thrombus. In certain patients with extensive iliofemoral DVT and no other co-morbidity at a low risk of bleeding, catheter-directed thrombolysis (CDT) can be used to reduce symptoms. CDT uses a catheter to deliver the thrombolytic agent directly to the clot, achieving a higher concentration of the drug at the site where it is needed, with a lower total dose than would be required with systemic thrombolytic therapy, which lowers the risk of intracranial haemorrhage (Vendantham *et al.* 2006). Balloon angioplasty and stent insertion is also carried out during CDT if obstruction is present. Thrombolytic therapy does not prevent clot propagation, rethrombosis or embolization, so oral anticoagulation therapy must also be initiated. The Society of Interventional Radiology found the incidence of PE following CDT to be 1% (less than the incidence of PE during standard anticoagulation therapy), with an 8% incidence of major bleeding. Further evidence needs to be collated, however, in a specific subgroup with iliofemoral DVT and limb-threatening disease, with a low bleeding risk; CDT shows a clinical benefit (Vendantham *et al.* 2006).

Inferior vena cava (IVC) filters

Indications for placement of an IVC include bleeding complications associated with anticoagulant therapy or any absolute contraindications to use of anticoagulants. Patients who develop recurrent VTE despite adequate anticoagulation can also be considered as candidates (Kearon *et al.* 1998). Historically, prior to the discovery of anticoagulation, DVT was treated by laparotomy and vena caval ligation, which results in high mortality rates. Treatment progressed onto the use of vena caval clips in an attempt to reduce the luminal diameter of the vessels to make clot propagation more difficult, and then onto the use of permanent filters. Filters aim to maintain caval patency, trap emboli, preserve prograde caval blood flow, avoid stasis and enhance the thrombolysis of trapped emboli. The current benchmark standard, in use for over 20 years, is the Greenfield filter, whose design achieves a long-term patency rate of 98% with only a 4% incidence of recurrent PE (Schreiber 2008).

Compression stockings

Elastic compression stockings with an ankle pressure gradient of 30–40 mmHg are recommended by the ACCP in patients with confirmed symptomatic DVT, alongside standard anticoagulation therapy, and should be continued for a minimum of two years (Kearon et al. 2008). Elastic stockings assist the calf muscle pump and reduce valvular reflux and venous hypertension, which contributes to the reduction of leg oedema and aids the microcirculation. Post-thrombotic syndrome affects almost 50% of patients with DVT. Regular use of compression stockings has been shown to reduce the incidence of this syndrome by 50% in compliant patients (Prandoni et al. 2004). Chapter 8 provides further detail.

Ambulation

Early ambulation (as tolerated) from day 2 after the initiation of out-patient anticoagulant therapy, in addition to effective compression, is strongly advised by the ACCP in patients with DVT. Early ambulation without compression stockings is not recommended. The fear of dislodging clots and precipitating a fatal PE is unfounded (Kearon et al. 2008).

Other treatments

Operative venous thrombectomy can be carried out to reduce acute symptoms and post-thrombotic mortality in selected patients with acute iliofemoral DVT if appropriate expertise and resources are available, although catheter-directed thrombolysis is preferred if patients have a low risk of bleeding. Postoperatively, patients should still receive anticoagulant therapy (Kearon et al. 2008).

Systemic thrombolytic therapy for DVT is not routinely used, but in patients with extensive proximal DVT who have a low risk of bleeding and where CDT is not available, systemic thrombolytic therapy can be used to reduce acute symptoms (Kearon et al. 2008).

Percutaneous mechanical thrombectomy is not recommended (Kearon et al. 2008).

Upper extremity DVT

Upper extremity DVT is the term commonly used to describe thrombosis of the axillary, brachial or subclavian veins. It is a relatively rare disorder, accounting for approximately 1–4% of all cases of DVT (Sajid *et al.* 2007) and thought to affect two per 100 000 people per year (Lindblad *et al.* 1988). Since it has the potential for significant mortality from PE, which is present in nearly one-third of these patients (Prandoni P *et al.* 1997), and there is no standardized therapy for upper extremity DVT, it will be discussed separately.

Upper extremity DVT can be classified as primary or secondary, depending on the cause. Primary upper extremity DVT is either idiopathic, in which case patients have no identifiable trigger for the thrombosis and no obvious underlying disease, or due to effort thrombosis, also referred to as Paget–Schroetter syndrome.

Patients with Paget–Schroetter syndrome are usually young and healthy and develop DVT, typically in their dominant arm, after strenuous exertion – during activities such as weight lifting, rowing or wrestling (Joffe *et al.* 2002). Physical exertion of the arm causes microtrauma to the intima of the vessel involved, which leads to activation of the coagulation cascade. Repeated insults to the wall of the vein can cause significant thrombosis, with eventual scar tissue formation, especially if there is a degree of mechanical compression upon the vessel, from thoracic outlet obstruction (Zell *et al.* 2001). Compression of the subclavian vein is often seen in athletes with hypertrophied muscles from heavy lifting, or in patients with cervical ribs or long transverse processes of the cervical spine (Joffe *et al.* 2002).

In those patients with idiopathic upper-extremity DVT, there has been an association with occult cancer. Girolami *et al.* (1999) found that one-quarter of people presenting with upper extremity DVT were diagnosed with cancer within 1 year of follow-up – typically lymphoma or lung cancer. The presence of hypercoagulable states in such patients is uncertain, due to varying results from observational studies. Screenings for coagulation disorders tend to produce results in patients who also have a family history of DVT, a history of recurrent unexplained pregnancy loss or prior DVT (Joffe *et al.* 2002).

Secondary thrombosis accounts for the majority of cases of upper extremity DVT and is described in patients with pacemakers or central venous catheters for chemotherapy, bone marrow transplantation, dialysis and parenteral nutrition. Up to one -quarter of patients with these indwelling devices develop upper extremity DVT (Horattas *et al.* 1988). Catheter related thrombi are caused by vessel wall damage during insertion or during infusion of medication and from impedance of blood flow through the vein, resulting in areas of venous stasis. Those patients with incorrectly placed venous catheters are more likely to develop thrombosis (Joffe *et al.* 2002).

Signs and symptoms

As with lower limb DVT, upper limb thrombi can be asymptomatic, especially if the axillary or subclavian veins are involved. More commonly shoulder or neck discomfort is reported, accompanied by arm oedema (Prandoni *et al.* 1997). If the superior vena cava becomes obstructed by the thrombus, patients will present with facial as well as arm oedema and may complain of blurred vision, vertigo and dyspnoea. If thoracic outlet obstruction occurs, patients may report pain in the forearm and the fourth and fifth digits, consistent with injury to the brachial plexus. Provocative tests can be performed to confirm such symptoms (see Box 5.3; Adson's and Wright's manoeuvres). Low-grade fever is often present and a reduced venous return to the heart as a result of superior vena caval obstruction can cause a sinus tachycardia. As with DVT in the lower limbs, a palpable cord may be felt and the affected limb may be cyanotic, with dilatation of the collateral veins over the arm and anterior chest wall. There is often jugular venous distension. Once again, these signs and symptoms are nonspecific and may occur in patients with lymphoedema, neoplastic compression of the blood vessels, haematoma, muscle injury or superficial vein thrombosis, therefore objective testing is required to determine the diagnosis.

Investigations

Non-invasive duplex ultrasonography is the imaging modality of choice when investigating for upper extremity DVT, as it has a high sensitivity and specificity. Shadowing from the clavicle, however, limits visualization of a short segment of the subclavian vein, which may result in a false-negative result (Haire *et al.* 1991). If practitioners suspect a clot despite a negative ultrasound, contrast venography may be required. It provides excellent visualization of the venous anatomy but requires the use of an intravenous contrast agent, which has its own associated risks and may worsen a pre-existing thrombus – not to mention the difficulty involved in cannulating a vein in the oedematous arm. If venography is not appropriate, magnetic resonance angiography (MRA) is an accurate and non-invasive method of thrombus detection but obviously cannot be used in patients with implanted metal (Hartnell *et al.* 1995).

Treatment

Treatment options for upper extremity DVT remain controversial, due to a lack of large randomized controlled trials and because the aetiology and prognosis can vary widely from patient to patient (Gaffar 2005). Options are outlined in Box 5.5. Simple measures, such as limb elevation and use of a graduated compression arm sleeve, can be combined with anticoagulation to maintain the patency of the collateral vessels and reduce thrombus propagation (Horattas 1988). Therapy is tailored to each individual patient; generally three months of warfarin therapy is recommended, with a target INR of 2–3 (with therapeutic doses of LMWH or UFH while this is being initiated, as described for lower limb DVT) (Kearon *et al.* 2008). Thrombolytic therapy is not

---

Box 5.5 Treatment options for upper extremity DVT

- *Limb elevation.*
- *Graduated compression arm sleeve.*
- *Anticoagulation* (see Chapter 7).
- *Catheter-directed thrombolysis* – image-guided therapy where thrombolytic agent is administered directly to the thrombus with catheter introduction. Balloon angioplasty and stents are also used to treat any underlying venous obstruction.
- *Suction thrombectomy* (or percutaneous mechanical thrombectomy) – involves catheter insertion to site of the thrombus, which is then removed. A variety of suction devices are in use.
- *Surgical thrombectomy* – involves open surgery to access the vein and completely remove the clot.
- *Angioplasty* – technique of mechanically widening an obstructed blood vessel by inflating a balloon-tipped catheter through the blockage, using imaging guidance.
- *Vein stenting* – may be performed with angioplasty; insertion of a small wire mesh tube in the vessel to help it to remain open.
- *Thoracic outlet decompression* – if conservative measures fail, Surgical intervention may involve removal of the scalene muscles, first rib or a cervial rib if present.
- *Superior vena cava filter* – insertion of a small metal basket to the superior vena cava to filter emboli passing through the bloodstream.

(Adapted from Joffe *et al.* 2002)

recommended routinely by the ACCP, due to a paucity of data surrounding its use. In studies carried out in the area thrombolytic therapy achieved success in terms of vessel patency, but in terms of clinical endpoints, such as PE occurrence, recurrent VTE, bleeding and post-thrombotic syndrome, it is not known how thrombolytic therapy compares to anticoagulant therapy (Kearon *et al.* 2008). In selected patients with severe symptoms and a low risk of bleeding, catheter-directed thrombolysis can achieve high rates of clot resolution with lower doses of medication, thus reducing the bleeding risk compared with systemic thrombolysis. Thrombolysis restores venous patency early, reducing the risk of long-term complications such as post-thrombotic syndrome. It is most effective in young, otherwise healthy patients with primary upper extremity DVT and those who require preservation of a mandatory central venous catheter (Kearon *et al.* 2008; Urschel *et al.* 2000).

Data on the effectiveness of surgical intervention is lacking. However, the studies that have been carried out show higher rates of vein patency and lower rates of post-thrombotic syndrome when surgery and lysis are combined (Machleder 1993). Any invasive procedure is associated with risks, and the benefits of surgical thrombectomy need to be evaluated against the risks of general anaesthesia and potential pneumothorax and brachial plexus injury. The ACCP therefore suggest that catheter extraction, surgical thrombectomy or transluminal angioplasty is reserved for patients in whom anticoagulant or thrombolytic treatment has failed (Kearon *et al.* 2008).

Surgical eradication of vein compression in upper extremity DVT has been shown to reduce the risk of recurrent thrombosis and complications in some studies (Hicken *et al.* 1998). For patients with thoracic outlet syndrome, a conservative approach, involving several months of physiotherapy to loosen the muscles compressing the subclavian vein, is advocated before surgical decompression is attempted (Parziale *et al.* 2000). Patients with primary upper extremity DVT are generally a younger, otherwise healthy population, therefore more aggressive treatment is advocated to reduce the risk of chronic venous insufficiency. In contrast, patients with secondary upper extremity DVT often have very high short-term mortality rates and most die from underlying medical problems, such as cancer or infection, rather than from the complications of their DVT (Hingorani *et al.* 1997). Conservative treatment with anticoagulation alone is therrefore generally recommended (Joffe 2002).

Patients in whom anticoagulation is contraindicated, or those patients who develop PE even with adequate anticoagulation, can be considered as candidates for placement of a superior vena cava (SVC) filter. Few trials have been completed regarding their use in upper extremity DVT and concerns regarding the risk of filter migration, dislodgment, fracture and precipitation of SVC syndrome have prevented their widespread use. In the small series of patients studied, they have been found to be protective against clinical PE (Ascher *et al.* 2000; Spence *et al.* 1999) and their use is recommended by the ACCP in selected patients who cannot tolerate anticoagulation and who have clinically significant PE or DVT progression (Kearon *et al.* 2008).

Complications

Complications of the condition include post-thrombotic syndrome (PTS) as a result of venous hypertension secondary to outflow obstruction and valvular damage, which can vary from mild oedema to incapacitating limb swelling with pain and ulceration (Joffe *et al.* 2002). Trials have shown the effectiveness of graduated compression stockings in reducing the rate of post-thrombotic syndrome in lower extremity DVT, but no controlled studies have evaluated their effectiveness in the upper extremities (Brandjes *et al.* 1997). Since anecdotal evidence suggests that patients may derive relief from such measures, elastic compression sleeves are recommended in symptomatic patients (Kearon *et al.* 2008). As well as PE, other complications of thrombus in the upper extremities include loss of vascular access, SVC syndrome, septic thrombophlebitis, thoracic duct obstruction and brachial plexopathy (Gaffar 2005). Lack of vascular access can prove particularly problematic in such patients. For patients who have upper extremity DVT associated with an indwelling central venous catheter, the ACCP recommend that the catheter remain *in situ* if it is functional and there remains an ongoing need for it to remain (Kearon *et al.* 2008).

Thrombosis in children

Compared to adult patients, the incidence of VTE is rare in children and there is still a paucity of evidence-based data available regarding the treatment of paediatric thrombosis; indeed, many of the guidelines for treatment in children are extrapolated from adult data (David *et al.* 1995). The prevalence of central and proximal venous thrombi that were previously undetected in children have increased, due to our abilities to detect such pathology using modern imaging techniques. Advances in the support given to critically ill children involving the widespread use of central venous catheters have also increased the incidence of DVT (Massicotte *et al.* 1998).

Rationale for antithrombotic therapy in children is the same as in adults. An important consideration in children is the impact thrombosis has on their long-term morbidity. PTS has been reported in 10–60% of children following VTE (Manco-Johnson 2006). Rapid restoration of venous patency might decrease the risk of PTS, and systemic thrombolytic therapy has been used successfully in children and should be considered in conjunction with a haematologist in children with high-risk clots, although further research into the area is required (Manco-Johnson 2006). In children with a first-episode VTE, UFH or LMWH can be safely used with monitoring of anti-factor Xa assays (Monagle *et al.* 2008). Neonates who experience VTE should have supportive care with radiological monitoring and subsequent anticoagulation if there is thrombus extension. Alternatively, anticoagulation can be started immediately if indicated based on a risk assessment of the child (Monagle *et al.* 2008).

VKAs are not popular in children but there are reports of successful treatment with warfarin from as early as the first week of life (Hartman *et al.* 1989). Warfarin adjustment requires close monitoring during infancy and children exhibit a high risk for exceeding their target INR. Oral anticoagulation with warfarin is usually started with a maintenance dose of 0.1 mg/kg, while heparin is continued until the INR reaches the target for two consecutive readings (Manco-Johnson 2006). Bleeding risk appears to be lower in children than for adults and reversal of anticoagulation is the same as in adults.

Courses of anticoagulants are usually finite in children, even if they are found to carry thrombophilic traits (Manco-Johnson 2006). If thrombosis is recurrent, there is a strong family history of recurrent VTE, there are three or more thrombophilic traits present or there is a persistently elevated D-dimer after 12 months of anticoagulation, then indefinite anticoagulation may be indicated (Manco-Johnson 2006). In addition to anticoagulation, compression stockings are recommended to prevent PTS, combined with nutritional and exercise advice to prevent obesity, which has been linked to the development of venous stasis ulcers (Manco-Johnson 2006).

Prophylaxis with UFH or LMWH can be given to children known to have thrombophilic traits during high-risk periods, such as perioperatively. Oestrogen-containing oral contraceptives are generally avoided in adolescents with antithrombin deficiency or the factor V Leiden mutation (Manco-Johnson 2006).

Case study 5.1: the footballer's sprain

A 60 year-old male lorry driver presents with a 3 day history of left calf discomfort. He played a game of five-a-side football the night before his symptoms started and thinks he might have 'sprained something'. Ibuprofen has not relieved the pain and now he feels his leg is tender to the touch, especially along the distribution of the major leg vessels, and appears slightly swollen. He is an overweight diet-controlled diabetic on no medications and has no other medical or family history of note. He smokes 20 cigarettes a day. You examine his left leg and find unilateral pitting oedema to mid-calf with a 2 cm difference in calf circumference between the right and left leg. He is afebrile and systemically well and you feel that the patient is likely to have a DVT.

Regarding Case Study 5.1, how would you proceed to investigate the man?

Follow a management algorithm as laid out in Figure 5.5. The patient's Wells score (see Table 5.1) has put him at medium-probability risk for DVT, D-dimer testing is bypassed and the patient has a lower limb ultrasound. If there is a delay in arranging the scan, then selected stable patients can avoid an overnight hospital admission and be given LMWH and asked to return for ultrasound the following day. DVT is confirmed and, after determining that he is at low risk of bleeding complications, it is decided to start the patient on warfarin therapy.

What advice would you provide?

The target of treatment is to achieve an INR that balances the therapeutic goal with the risk of bleeding on an individual basis. High loading doses of warfarin are no longer recommended and current advice is to start treatment closer to the maintenance dose expected to be used. Consider potential drug interactions based on what medication the patient takes (in this case nothing). Make sure to ask about herbal remedies and over-the-counter supplements. Start with an initial daily dose of 5 mg, aiming for a target INR of 2–3. Avoid frequent dose adjustments, bearing in mind that a change in dose can take >48 hours to influence the INR. INR monitoring should be started after the initial two or three doses and then every other day during initiation. INR is then measured less frequently, depending on the response of the patient. Once a steady state is reached, most patients remain well controlled with 4–6 weekly testing and dose adjustment. All patients should be educated on why the treatment is indicated:

- Mechanism of action of warfarin.
- Ensuring the patient understands the need to take it at the same time each time.
- INR – the need for regular testing and the target range.
- Signs and symptoms of bleeding.
- How warfarin can be effected by alcohol, common over-the-counter medications, an excess of vitamin K-rich foods and any concurrent illnesses.
- The need to alert other health professionals to being on the medication prior to any invasive procedures, surgery or dental work.

Chapter 7 provides further information on initiation of warfarin.

Conclusion

This chapter has provided a complete overview of the signs, symptoms and differential diagnoses of DVT, including the rarer presentation of upper extremity DVT and thrombosis in children. After reading this chapter you should have an awareness of the use of clinical prediction tools and how they can aid in the choice of appropriate investigations. Treatment options have been discussed; however, Chapter 7 has been dedicated to the topic of anticoagulation.

References

American Thoracic Society (ATS) (1999) The diagnostic approach to acute venous thromboembolism. Clinical practice guideline. *American Journal of Respiratory and Critical Care Medicine* **160**: 1043–1066.

Ascher E, Hingorani A, Tsemekhin B *et al.* (2000) Lessons learned from a 6-year clinical experience with superior vena cava Greenfield filters. *Journal of Vascular Surgery* **32**: 881–887.

Barham K, Shah T (2007) Images in clinical medicine: phlegmasia cerulea dolens. *New England Journal of Medicine* **356**: 3.

Belcaro G, Nicolaides AN, Errichi BM *et al.* (1999) Superficial thrombophlebitis of the legs: a randomised, controlled, follow up study. *Angiology* **50**: 523–529.

Belch JJF, McMillan NC, Fogelman I *et al.* (1981) Combined phlebography and arthrography in patients with painful swollen calf. *British Medical Journal* **282**: 949.

Bergqvist D, Jaroszewski H (1986) Deep vein thrombosis in patients with superficial thrombophlebitis of the leg. *British Medical Journal* **292**: 658.

Bersier DE, Bounameaux H (2003) Cellulitis and deep vein thrombosis: a controversial association. *Journal of Thrombosis and Haemostasis* **1**: 867–868.

Blann AD, Lip GYH (2006) Venous thromboembolism. *British Medical Journal* **332**: 215–219.

Borgstede JP, Clagett GE (1992) Types, frequency and significance of alternative diagnoses found during duplex Doppler venous examinations of the lower extremities. *Journal of Ultrasound Medicine* **11**: 85–89.

Bounameaux H, de Moerloose P, Perrier A (1994) Plasma measurements of D-dimer as a diagnostic aid in suspected venous thromboembolism. *Thrombosis and Haemostasis* **71**: 1–6.

Brandjes DPM, Buller HR, Heijboer H *et al.* (1997) Randomised trial of the effect of compression stockings in patients with symptomatic proximal vein thrombosis. *Lancet* **349**: 759–762.

Browse NL, Burnand KG, Thomas ML (1988) Deep vein thrombosis: diagnosis. In *Diseases of the Veins: Pathology, Diagnosis and Treatment*, 1st Edition. Arnold, London.

Cogo, A, Lensing, AWA, Prins, MH, *et al.* (1998) Compression ultrasonography for diagnostic management of patients with clinically suspected deep vein thrombosis: prospective cohort study. *British Medical Journal* **316**: 17–20.

David M, Manco-Johnson M, Andrew M (1995) Diagnosis and treatment of venous thromboembolism in children and adolescents. *Thrombosis and Haemostasis* **74**: 791–792.

Diehm C, Allenberg JR, Nimura-Eckert K *et al.* (2000) Diseases of veins. In *Color Atlas of Vascular Diseases*, 1st Edition. Springer-Verlag, Milan.

Erdman WA, Jayson HT, Redman HC *et al.* (1990) Deep venous thrombosis of the extremities: role of MRI in the diagnosis. *Radiology* **174**: 425–431.

Feied C (2005) Deep venous thrombosis. eMedicine: http://www.emedicine.com/MED/topic2785.htm

Flanc C, Kakkar VV, Clark MB (1968) The detection of venous thrombosis of the legs using ^{125}I labelled fibrinogen. *British Journal of Surgery* **55**: 742.

Gaffar M (2005) Upper-extremity deep vein thrombosis. *Hospital Physician* **29–34**. Available at: http://www.turner-white.com/memberfile.php?PubCode=hp_jun05_vein.pdf

Girolami A, Prandoni P, Zanon E *et al.* (1999) Venous thromboses of upper limbs are more frequently associated with occult cancer as compared with those of lower limbs. *Blood Coagulation Fibrinolysis* **10**: 455–457.

Gorman PW, Davis KR, Donnelly R (2000) ABC of arterial and venous disease: Swollen lower limb – 1: general assessment and deep vein thrombosis. *British Medical Journal* **320**: 1453–1456.

Haire WD, Lynch TG, Lund GB *et al.* (1991) Limitations of magnetic resonance imaging and ultrasound directed (duplex) scanning in the diagnosis of subclavian vein thrombosis. *Journal of Vascular Surgery* **13**: 391–397.

Hartman KR, Manco-Johnson M, Rawlings JS *et al.* (1989) Homozygous protein c deficiency: early treatment with warfarin. *American Journal of Pediatric Hematology and Oncology* **11**: 395–401.

Hartnell GG, Hughes LA, Finn JP *et al.* (1995) Magnetic resonance angiography of the central chest veins: a new gold standard? *Chest* **107**: 1053–1057.

Hassan TB (2000) Clinical decision units in the emergency department: old concepts, new paradigms, and refined gate keeping. *Emergency Medicine Journal* **20**: 123–125.

Havig O (1977) Deep vein thrombosis and pulmonary embolism. An autopsy study with multiple regression analysis of possible risk factors. *Acta Chirurgica Scandinavica Supplementum* **478**: 1–120.

Heijboer H, Jongbloets LM, Buller HR *et al.* (1992) The clinical utility of real time compression ultrasonography in the diagnostic management of patients with recurrent venous thrombosis. *Acta Radiologica Scandinavica* **33**: 297–300.

Hicken GJ, Ameli M (1998) Management of subclavian axillary vein thrombosis: a review. *Canadian Journal of Surgery* **41**: 13–25.

Hingorani A, Ascher E, Lorenson E *et al.* (1997) Upper extremity deep venous thrombosis and its impact on morbidity and mortality rates in a hospital based population. *Journal of Vascular Surgery* **26**: 853–860.

Hirsh J, Hull RD, Raskob GE (1986) Clinical features and diagnosis of venous thrombosis. *Journal of the American College of Cardiologists* **8**: 114–127B.

Homans J (1928) Thrombophlebitis of the lower extremities. *Annals of Surgery* **88**: 641.

Horattas MC, Wright DJ, Fenton AH *et al.* (1988) Changing concepts of deep venous thrombosis of the upper extremity: report of a series and review of the literature. *Surgery* **104**: 561–567.

Joffe HV, Goldhaber SZ (2002) Upper-extremity deep vein thrombosis. *Circulation* **106**: 1874–1880.

Kakkar VV, Howe CT, Nicolaides AN, Renney JTG, Clarke MB (1970) Deep vein thrombosis of the leg- is there a high risk group. *American Journal of Surgery* **120**: 527–530.

Kearon C, Julian JA, Newman TE *et al.*(1998a) Noninvasive diagnosis of deep vein thrombosis. *Annals of Internal Medicine* **128**: 663–677

Kearon C, Ginsberg JS, Hirsch J (1998b) The role of venous ultrasonography in the diagnosis of suspected deep venous thrombosis and pulmonary embolism. *Annals of Internal Medicine* **129**: 1044–1049.

Kearon C, Ginsberg JS, Douketis J *et al.* (2001) Management of suspected deep venous thrombosis in outpatients by using clinical assessment and D-dimer testing. *Annals of Internal Medicine* **135**: 108–111.

Kearon C, Kahn SR, Agnelli G *et al.* (2008) Antithrombotic therapy for venous thromboembolic disease: American College of Chest Physicians evidence based clinical practice guidelines, 8th Edition. *Chest* **133**: 454–545

Kelly J, Hunt BJ (2002a) Role of D-dimers in diagnosis of venous thromboembolism. *Lancet* **359**: 456–457.

Kelly J, Rudd A, Lewis RR *et al.* (2002b) Plasma D-dimers in the diagnosis of venous thromboembolism. *Archives of Internal Medicine* **162**: 747–756.

Lindblad B, Tengborn L, Bergqvist D (1988) Deep vein thrombosis of the axillary-subclavian veins: epidemiologic data, effects of different types of treatment and late sequelae. *European Journal of Vascular Surgery* **2**: 161–165.

Lucia MA, Ely EW (2001) Images in clinical medicine superficial thrombophlebitis. *New England Journal of Medicine* **19;344**(16): 1214.

Machleder HI (1993) Evaluation of a new treatment strategy for Paget–Schroetter syndrome: spontaneous thrombosis of the axillary–subclavian vein. *Journal of Vascular Surgery* **17**: 305–317.

Makin GS (1968) Assessment of a simple test to detect postoperative deep vein thrombosis. *British Journal of Surgery* **55**: 822.

Manco-Johnson MJ (2006) How I treat venous thrombosis in children. *Blood* **107**: 21–29.

Massicotte MP, Dix D, Monagle P *et al.* (1998) Central venous catheter related thrombosis in children: analysis of the Canadian registry of venous thromboembolic complications. *Journal of Pediatrics* **133**: 770–776.

McFarlane DG, Bacon PA (1980) Popliteal cyst rupture in normal knee joints. *British Medical Journal* **281**: 1203.

McLachlin J, Richards T, Paterson JC (1962) An evaluation of clinical signs in the diagnosis of venous thrombosis. *Archives of Surgery* **85**: 738.

Monagle P, Chalmers E, Chan A (2008) Antithrombotic therapy in neonates and children. *Chest* **133**: 887–968S.

Murphy TP, Cronan JJ (1990) Evolution of deep vein thrombosis: a propspective evaluation with ultrasound. *Radiology* **177**: 543–548.

Neale D, Tovey C, Vali A *et al.* (2004) Evaluation of the Simplify D-dimer assay as a screening test for the diagnosis of deep vein thrombosis in an emergency department. *Emergency Medicine Journal* **21**: 663–666.

O'Donnell TF Jr, Abbott WM, Athanasoulis CA *et al.* (1980) Diagnosis of deep vein thrombosis in the outpatient by venography. *Surgery Gynecology and Obstetrics* **150**: 69–74.

Palareti G, Legnani C, Cosmi B *et al.* (2002) Risk of venous thromboembolism recurrence: high negative predictive value of D-dimer performed after oral anticoagulation is stopped. *Thrombosis and Hemostasis* **87**: 7–12.

Palareti G, Cosmi B, Legani C *et al.* (2006) D-dimer testing to determine the duration of anticoagulation therapy. *New England Journal of Medicine* **355**: 1780–1789.

Parziale JR, Akelman E, Weiss AP *et al.* (2000) Thoracic outlet syndrome. *American Journal of Orthopedics* **29**: 353–360.

Perrier A, Desmarais S, Miron M *et al.* (1999) Non-invasive diagnosis of venous thromboembolism in outpatients. *Lancet* **353**: 190–195.

Poulose K, Kapcar A, Reba R (1976) False positive ^{125}I fibrinogen test. *Angiology* **27**: 258.

Prandoni P, Polistena P, Bernardi E *et al.* (1997) Upper-extremity deep vein thrombosis: risk factors, diagnosis and complications. *Archives of Internal Medicine* **157**: 57–62.

Prandoni P, Lensing AW, Prins MH *et al.* (2004) Below knee elastic compression stockings to prevent post-thrombotic syndrome: a randomized, controlled trial. *Annals of Internal Medicine* **141**: 249–256.

Rabinov K, Paulin S (1972) Roentgen diagnosis of venous thrombosis in the leg. *Archives of Surgery* **104**: 134–144.

Ramzi, DW, Leeper KV (2004) DVT and pulmonary embolism: part I. Diagnosis. *American Family Physician* **69**: 2829–2836.

Ross MA, Graff LG (2001) Principles of observation medicine. *Emergency Medicine Clinics of North America* **19**: 1–15.

Sadosty AT, Goyal DG, Boie ET *et al.* (2001) Emergency department D-dimer testing. *Journal of Emergency Medicine* **21**: 423–429.

Sajid MS, Ahmed N, Desai M *et al.* (2007) Upper limb deep vein thrombosis: a literature review to streamline the protocol for management. *Acta Haematologica* **118**: 10–18.

Sandler DA, Duncan JS, Ward P *et al.* (1984) Diagnosis of deep vein thrombosis: comparison of clinical evaluation, ultrasound, plethysmography and venoscan with X-ray venogram. *Lancet* **2**: 716–718.

Scarvelis D, Wells PS (2006) Diagnosis and treatment of deep-vein thrombosis. *Canadian Medical Association Journal* **175**: 1087–1092.

Schreiber D (2008) Deep venous thrombosis and thrombophlebitis. Emedicine. Available at: http://www.emedicine.medscape.com/article/758140 (last accessed 11 January 2009)

Simpson FG, Robinson PJ, Bark M *et al.* (1980) Prospective study of thrombophlebitis and 'pseudothrombophlebitis'. *Lancet* **1**: 331.

Spence LD, Gironta MG, Malde H *et al.* (1999) Acute upper extremity deep venous thrombosis: safety and effectiveness of superior vena caval filters. *Radiology* **210**: 53–58.

Swarczinski C, Dijkers M (1991) The value of serial leg measurements for monitoring deep vein thrombosis in spinal cord injury. *Journal of Neuroscience Nursing* **23**: 306–314.

Tovey C, Wyatt S (2003) Diagnosis, investigation, and management of deep vein thrombosis. *British Medical Journal* **326**: 1180–1184.

Urschel HC, Razzuk MA (2000) Paget–Schroetter syndrome: what is the best management? *Annals of Thoracic Surgery* **69**: 1663–1669.

Van Dongen CJ, Van den Belt AG, Prins MH *et al.* (2004) Fixed dose subcutaneous low molecular weight heparin versus adjusted dose unfractionated heparin for venous thromboembolism [review]. *Cochrane Database Systematic Review*: CD001100.

Vendantham S, Milward SF, Cardella JF *et al.* (2006) Society of Interventional Radiology position statement: treatment of acute iliofemoral deep vein thrombosis with use of adjunctive catheter-directed intrathrombus thrombolysis. *Journal of Vascular Interventional Radiology* **17**: 613–616.

Verhovsek M, Douketis JD, Yi Q *et al.* (2008) Systematic review: D-dimer to predict recurrent disease after stopping anticoagulant therapy for unprovoked venous thromboembolism. *Annals of Internal Medicine* **149**: 481–490.

Wells PS, Lensing AWA, Davidson BL *et al.* (1995a) Accuracy of ultrasound for the diagnosis of deep vein thrombosis in asymptomatic patients after orthopaedic surgery. A meta-analysis. *Annals of Internal Medicine* **122**: 47–53.

Wells PS, Anderson DR, Bormanis J *et al.* (1997) Value of assessment of pre-test probability of deep-vein thrombosis in clinical management. *Lancet* **350**: 1795–1798.

Wells PS, Hirsch J, Anderson DR *et al.* (1998) A simple clinical model for the diagnosis of deep vein thrombosis combined with impedence plethysmography: potential for an improvement in the diagnostic process. *Journal of Internal Medicine* **243**: 15–23.

Wells PS, Anderson DR (2000) Diagnosis of deep-vein thrombosis in the year 2000. *Current Opinions in Pulmonary Medicine* **6**: 309–313.

Wells PS, Hirsh J, Anderson DR *et al.* (1995) Accuracy of clinical assessment of deep-vein thrombosis. *Lancet* **345**: 1326–1330.

Wheeler HB (1985) Diagnosis of deep venous thrombosis: review of clinical evaluation and impedance plethysmography. *American Journal of Surgery* **150**: 7–13.

Zell L, Kindermann W, Marschall F *et al.* (2001) Paget–Schroetter syndrome in sports activities: case study and literature review. *Angiology* **52**: 337–342.

Pulmonary embolism

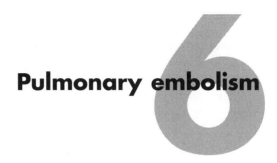

Overview

Just like DVT, the diagnosis of PE cannot be reliably made based on clinical acumen alone. Fatal PE is often undiagnosed even when a patient has recently seen a physician (Pineda *et al.* 2001). This has been proved by autopsy studies in which patients were found to have PE which had been missed ante mortem (Lindblad *et al.* 1991; Goldhaber *et al.* 1982).

Suspicion of the condition based on clinical findings and the presence of risk factors should be combined with thorough investigation to reach a conclusion. A negative D-dimer in patients of low or intermediate clinical probability reliably excludes PE, and further imaging is not required. When indicated, computed tomography pulmonary angiogram (CTPA) is the imaging test of choice. Lung isotope scanning is widely used in selected patients, depending on hospital facilities, but a non-diagnostic result must always be followed by further imaging.

The management of acute massive PE differs from the way a non-massive PE is handled. Thrombolysis is the first-line treatment for massive PE but not for non-massive PE – heparin is used

Venous Thromboembolism: A Nurses Guide to Prevention and Management By Ellen Welch
© 2010 John Wiley & Sons, Ltd.

[preferably low molecular weight heparin (LMWH)] and oral anticoagulation is commenced once VTE is reliably confirmed. Testing for thrombophilia is suggested in patients aged under 50 with recurrent VTE and a strong family history, but investigations for occult cancer should only be done if clinically suspected.

This chapter explores the condition in further detail.

Signs and symptoms

The clinical manifestations of PE are caused by strain upon the heart and lungs due to the presence of the clot in the lungs' circulation, and presentation can vary from sudden catastrophic circulatory collapse to gradually progressive dyspnoea (BTS 2003). Cardiac arrest is the most extreme presentation, occurring in 2% of patients with PE, usually from immediate asystole or pulseless electrical activity (Courtney DM *et al.* 2001).

The most common symptoms of PE in the PIOPED study were dyspnoea (73%), pleuritic chest pain (66%), cough (37%) and haemoptysis (13%) (PIOPED 1990). Atypical symptoms can also include fever, wheezing and chest wall pain (Tapson 2008) (see Table 6.1).

It is useful to divide the presentation of PE into four groups, based on the severity of presentation:

1. *Massive PE.* The patient has an embolus large enough to compromise the pulmonary circulation, which results in shock. The patient is hypotensive, pale, sweaty, oliguric and often drowsy due to poor perfusion. Tachycardia and tachypnoea are present. Signs of pulmonary hypertension may be evident, such as elevated neck veins, a loud P2, a right ventricular S3 gallop and a systolic murmur indicative of tricuspid regurgitation (Tapson 2008). Suggestive ECG changes are often present in this group, accompanied by hypoxia on arterial blood gas (ABG) analysis, and echocardiography will typically show features of right heart strain (BTS 2003).

2. *Acute pulmonary infarction.* This manifests with acute onset of pleuritic chest pain, breathlessness and often haemoptysis. Pain may be similar to ischaemic myocardial pain but will show no response to nitroglycerine, and ECG should help to distinguish the two. Examination can often show signs of pleural effusion, pleural friction rub and even localized chest wall tenderness.

Table 6.1 Frequency of signs and symptoms in patients at risk for PE

	PE confirmed (%) (PIOPED study, n = 117)	PE ruled out (%) (PIOPED study, n = 248)
Symptoms		
Dyspnoea	73	72
Pleuritic chest pain	66	59
Cough	37	36
Leg pain	26	24
Haemoptysis	13	8
Palpitations	10	18
Wheezing	9	11
Anginal pain	4	6
Signs		
Respiratory rate >20 per minute	70	68
Crackles	51	40
Heart rate >100 beats per minute	30	24
Fourth heart sound	24	13
Accentuated pulmonary component of second heart sound	23	13
Temperature >38.5 °C	7	12
Homans' sign	4	2
Pleural friction rub	3	2
Third heart sound	3	4
Cyanosis	1	2

[Data from PIOPED study (Stein *et al.* 1991)]

3. *Acute embolism without infarction.* Patients have non-specific symptoms of dyspnoea and/or chest discomfort accompanied by non-specific physical signs that could easily be secondary to another disease process. Tachypnoea and tachycardia are frequently present and occasionally crackles may be heard in the area of embolization.

4. *Multiple pulmonary emboli.* This group consists of patients who have repeated documented episodes of PE over several years and eventually present with signs and symptoms of pulmonary hyper-

tension and cor pulmonale. It also includes patients who have no previous documented episodes of PE but are found to have widespread obstruction of the pulmonary vessels with clots, presenting with gradually progressive dyspnoea, intermittent exertional chest pain and, eventually, features of pulmonary hypertension and cor pulmonale (Robinson 2006).

Investigations

As with DVT, PE cannot be diagnosed with certainty based on history and examination alone, and the list of differential diagnoses is immense (Box 6.1). A number of investigations are at our disposal to facilitate diagnosis. First-line investigations performed include electrocardiogram, chest radiography and arterial blood gas measurements, all of which can assist in ruling out other causes of the presenting symptoms. D-dimer blood testing can be carried out in conjunction with a pretest clinical probability assessment, the results of which can guide clinicians to decide whether further imaging is required to confirm the diagnosis.

Box 6.1 Differential diagnosis of PE

The list is extensive. An alternative diagnosis should be confirmed, or PE excluded before discontinuing the work-up:

- Acute coronary syndrome.
- Anaemia.
- Aortic stenosis.
- Atrial fibrillation.
- Cardiogenic shock.
- Chronic obstructive pulmonary disease.
- Cor pulmonale.
- Costochondritis.
- Herpes zoster.
- Hyperventilation.
- Mitral stenosis.
- Musculoskeletal pain.
- Myocarditis.
- Pericarditis.
- Pleuritis.
- Pneumonia.
- Pneumothorax.
- Rib fracture.
- Salicylate intoxication.
- Septic shock.
- Sudden cardiac death.
- Syncope.
- Toxic shock syndrome.

(Adapted from Sharma 2006)

Pretest probability assessment

As with DVT, it is good practice to use clinical prediction rules to establish the likelihood of a diagnosis of PE. The Geneva score (Table 6.2) is such a protocol, however, the most widely implemented scoring system at use in the UK is based on criteria suggested by a Canadian group (BTS 2003, Wells PS *et al.* 2000). Known as Wells criteria it requires the patient to have clinical featurs compatible with PE combined with two other factors – the presence of a major risk factor and the absence of another clinical explanation (see Table 6.3).

Haemodynamically stable patients who present to the Emergency Department (ED) with suspected PE may be candidates for rapid investigation on a clinical decisions unit within the ED. The Leeds Teaching Hospital NHS Trust has developed a comprehensive protocol for such patients, combining a thorough clinical evaluation to exclude alterna-

Table 6.2 The Geneva score

Criterion	Points value
Age	
60–79	+1
>80	+2
Previous DVT/PE	+2
Recent surgery (<4 weeks ago)	+3
Heart rate >100 bpm	+1
$PaCO_2$	
<35 mmHg (4.6 kPa)	+2
35–39 mmHg (4.6–5.19 kPa)	+1
PaO_2	
<49 mmHg (6.52 kPa)	+4
49–59 mmHg (6.52–7.85 kPa)	+3
60–71 mmHg (7.98–9.44 kPa)	+2
72–82 (9.58–10.91 kPa)	+1
CXR	
Band atelectasis	+1
Elevation of hemidiaphragm	+1

Total score: <5, low probability of PE; 5–8, moderate probability of PE; >8, high probability of PE

Table 6.3 The Wells score used at The Leeds Teaching Hospitals NHS trust

Criterion	Points value
Clinical signs of DVT	+3
Alternative diagnosis less probable than PE	+3
Heart rate >100 bpm	+1.5
Immobilization or surgery <4 weeks ago	+1.5
Previous DVT/PE	+1.5
Haemoptysis	+1
Cancer	+1

Total score: <2, low probability of PE; 2–6, moderate probability of PE; >6, high probability of PE.
Reproduced with permission from The Leeds Hospital Trust Clinical decisions unit protocol (adapted from Wells *et al.* 2000).

tive diagnoses using a Well's score and appropriate investigations (see Figure 6.1). The flowchart also incorporates an assessment of patient suitability for outpatient 'ambulatory care', which allows selected low-risk patients to be appropriately investigated while avoiding a hospital stay.

Electrocardiography (ECG)

ECG changes in the setting of PE are generally quite non-specific and include T-wave changes, ST segment abnormalities, right bundle branch block (RBBB) and axis deviation (for further information regarding ECG interpretation please refer to a textbook focused on this topic). Sinus tachycardia is the most common finding and the 'classic' S1 Q3 T3 pattern typically described in PE is a rare finding (Robinson 2006). ECG changes are detectable when the PE is big enough to disturb right ventricular function. Large emboli increase right-sided afterload, causing pulmonary hypertension. The S1Q3T3 pattern reflects this right ventricular strain (Figure 6.2).

If the right ventricle enlarges the interventricular septum will deviate to the left, which stretches the right bundle branch, thus causing RBBB. A large clinical trial conducted among large numbers of patients with proven PE showed that 32% of patients with massive PE have manifestations of acute cor pulmonale on the ECG (S1 Q3 T3 pattern, RBBB, P-wave pulmonale or right axis deviation) (Anonymous, 1973). The low frequency of specific ECG changes associated with PE was con-

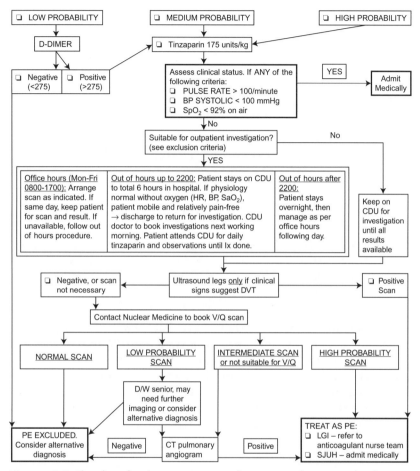

Figure 6.1 Flowchart for the management of patients with suspected pulmonary embolus. Reproduced with permission from the Leeds Teaching Hospitals Trust.

firmed by the Prospective Investigation of Pulmonary Embolism Diagnosis study (PIOPED 1990).

Arterial blood gas (ABG) analysis

Hypoxaemia is common in acute PE, but a normal PaO_2 may sometimes provide a false sense of security. Young patients without underlying lung disease may be able to compensate even with a PE and so may have a normal PaO_2 on ABG analysis [American Thoracic Society (ATS) 1999]. In a study of ABG results in patients with proven PE, the

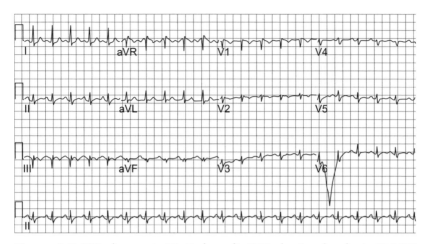

Figure 6.2 ECG changes in PE. Tachycardic ECG showing the classic S1Q3T3 pattern. ECG is showing a prominent S wave in lead I, a Q wave in lead III and an inverted T wave in lead III.

PaO_2 was found to vary according to age. PaO_2 was >80 mmHg in 29% of patients under 40 years of age, compared with 3% in the older age groups (Green *et al.* 1992). The alveolar–arterial oxygen tension difference was found to be abnormally elevated by more than 20 mmHg in 86% of patients with PE (Stein *et al.* 1991). Profound hypoxia with a normal chest radiograph in the absence of pre-existing lung disease is highly suggestive of pulmonary thromboembolism.

Chest radiology

Chest X-ray (CXR) findings in PE are generally nonspecific. Common findings include atelectasis, pulmonary infiltrates and evidence of an elevated hemidiaphragm (Stein *et al.* 1991). The presence of a pleural effusion increases the likelihood of PE in young patients who present with acute pleuritic chest pain (McNeill *et al.* 1976). Classic radiographic findings include 'Hampton's hump', the name given to areas of pulmonary infarction visible on the CXR, and 'Westermark's sign', areas of decreased vascularity (Figure 6.3). Such signs are suggestive of PE but are found infrequently. The CXR cannot be relied upon to prove or exclude PE; it is useful for the diagnosis of pneumonia or pneumothorax but it is important to remember that PE may coexist with these other conditions. A normal CXR in the setting of severe dyspnoea without evidence of bronchospasm or a cardiac shunt is strongly suggestive of PE (ATS 1999).

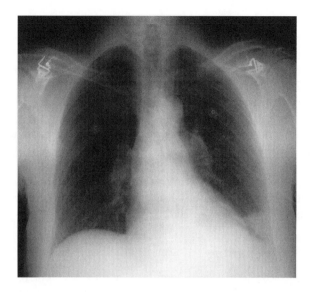

Figure 6.3 Chest X-ray (CXR) changes in PE. CXR demonstrating a pleural-based wedge-shaped pulmonary infarction at the left lung base (Hampton's hump), with focal avascularity in the right upper lung field (Westermark's sign). This patient had multiple PE. From Sokolove PE, Offerman SR (2001) Pulmonary embolism. *New England Journal of Medicine* **345**: 1311. Copyright © 2007, Massachusetts Medical Society. All rights reserved.

D-dimer

D-dimers are released as a result of fibrinolysis and indicate the presence of an intravascular thrombus, as outlined in Chapter 5. The test is only useful in excluding PE and should only be used in combination with a pretest probability assessment. A negative D-dimer reliably excludes PE in patients with a low pretest probability. A positive or intermediate result warrants further investigation. The longer a patient has been in hospital, the more likely for D-dimer testing to produce false positives, due to clot formation at venepuncture sites, and venous stasis, due to bed rest (Robinson 2006).

Patients with a high pretest probability who you know are going to require further investigations should not have a D-dimer test. Inappropriate testing has economic impacts and subjects the patient to unnecessary venepuncture (Fiappo *et al.* 2009).

Cardiac troponin

Troponin is a protein found in cardiac and skeletal muscle. Certain subtypes are very sensitive indicators of damage to heart muscle and are routinely used as markers of myocardial damage in patients with acute coronary syndromes.

Recent studies have shown that right heart strain in massive PE can be detected by the release of cardiac troponins (Giannitsis *et al.* 2000; Douketis 2002; Janata *et al.* 2003). This is due to the damage to the muscular right ventricle (Iwadate *et al.* 2001). The degree of right ventricular strain has been shown to affect outcome post-PE – one study showed that 1 year mortality from PE was 13% in the presence of right ventricular afterload stress detected by echocardiography, compared to 1.3% without (Kasper *et al.* 1997). Troponin measurements may therefore be helpful in providing prognostic information but the role of troponin in diagnosing PE is limited, since it will not be released in non-massive PE (Dieter *et al.* 2002).

Isotope lung scanning

Isotope lung scanning is also known as ventilation–perfusion (V/Q) scanning. The V/Q scan was historically the pivotal diagnostic test in acute PE until several studies confirmed its lack of reliability (PIOPED Investigators 1990; Nilsson *et al.* 2001; Prologo *et al.* 2002). The test uses radioactive contrast material to evaluate areas of ventilation in the lungs compared with areas of regional lung blood flow. Patients are asked to inhale small doses of a nebulized radioactive material, after which the lungs are imaged. Intravenous (i.v.) radioactive contrast is then given and further images are taken to assess blood flow to the lungs. If a PE is present, there will be reduced perfusion to the segment of lung affected but lung ventilation will be normal (Figure 6.4) (British Nuclear Medicine Society 2003). Details regarding appropriate techniques for isotope lung scanning are available elsewhere (Stein *et al.* 1974).

There is no consistent terminology in use for reporting and results are generally reported as either a low, intermediate or high probability for PE (BTS 2003), which can lead to erroneous interpretation of the results (Bastuji-Garin *et al.* 1998). Modified criteria for the interpretation of V/Q scans are shown in Table 6.4. Most lung diseases affect pulmonary blood flow and ventilation to some extent, which reduces the specificity of the V/Q scan (McNeil 1976; Velchik *et al.* 1989; Newman *et al.* 1972). It is commonly concluded that a high-probability lung scan is diagnostic of PE, but the PIOPED investigators and other researchers since then have shown that false positives occur in patients with previous PE (Van Beek *et al.* 2001). More importantly, the PIOPED study determined that PE is often present in patients with a non-diagnostic lung scan when associated with a high clinical suspicion of PE. In this

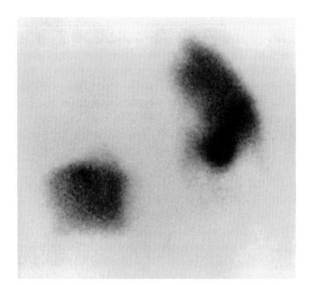

Figure 6.4 Ventilation/perfusion (VQ) scan. VQ scan taken from the same patient X-rayed in Figure 6.2. Scan showed normal ventilation images but loss of perfusion to the entire right upper lobe as well as to the anterior, lateral and medial basal segments of the left lower lobe. From Sokolove PE, Offerman SR (2001). Pulmonary embolism. *New England Journal of Medicine* **345**: 1311. Copyright © 2007, Massachusetts Medical Society. All rights reserved.

Table 6.4 Modified PIOPED criteria for interpretation of V/Q scans

Probability	Criteria
High	>1 large V/Q mismatch
	1 Large plus >1 moderate V/Q mismatch
	>3 Moderate V/Q mismatch
Intermediate (indeterminate)	1 Large V/Q mismatch
	<4 Moderate V/Q mismatch
	1 Matched V/Q defect plus normal CXR
Low	1 V/Q mismatch plus normal chest radiograph
	>1 Matched V/Q defects plus some normal Q plus normal CXR
	Small Q defects plus normal CXR
	Non-segmental Q defects (such as small pleural effusion, cardiomegaly, enlarged mediastinal structures, raised hemidiaphragm)
Normal	No Q defects present; Q exactly outlines the shape of the lungs on CXR

V, ventilation; Q, perfusion; CXR, chest X-ray.
(PIOPED Investigators, 1990) (BTS 1997) reproduced with permission from the BMJ group.

setting, a high-probability scan is associated with proven PE in 96% of cases, but a low-probability scan is associated with PE in 40% (ATS 1999). An indeterminate result is also commonplace in elderly patients (Righini *et al.* 2000) and in those with chronic airways disease, cardiopulmonary disease or any condition that causes intrapulmonary shadowing on the CXR, and these patients often go on to require further imaging (Hartmann *et al.* 2000). In subjects undergoing investigation for PE, an abnormal CXR increases the prevalence of non-diagnostic V/Q scans, whereas a normal pretest CXR is more often associated with a definitive result (i.e. normal or high probability) (Forbes *et al.* 2001).

The BTS have concluded that isotope lung scanning can be considered as the initial imaging of choice in the diagnosis of PE, provided that: the CXR is normal; there is no significant symptomatic concurrent cardiopulmonary disease; standard reporting criteria are used; and a non-diagnostic result is always followed by further imaging. Over one-third of District General Hospitals in the United Kingdom do not have access to isotope lung scanning on site (Burkill *et al.* 1999), leading the BTS to add a further stipulation that lung scanning only be used as a first-line measure if the hospital has the facilities to carry it out on site. Where isotope lung scanning is normal, PE is reliably excluded –but a significant minority of high-probability results are false positives (BTS 2003).

Lower extremity studies

Over 70% of cases of fatal or non-fatal proven PE have proximal DVT, even though this is typically asymptomatic (Bergqvist *et al.* 1985; Saeger *et al.* 1994; Hull *et al.* 1983). Half of those with proximal DVT have concurrent PE (Monreal *et al.* 1992; Dorfman *et al.* 1987). In cases where lung scanning is non-diagnostic of PE, evaluating the lower extremities for evidence of DVT can determine the need for anticoagulation. If ultrasound is positive, then treatment can be initiated without needing to expose the patient to further, more invasive and more expensive investigations. As mentioned in Chapter 3, colour-flow Doppler imaging combined with compression ultrasonography has a high sensitivity and specificity (89–100%) for detection of proximal DVT in symptomatic patients. It is not as sensitive (33–58%) in patients without symptoms of DVT (ATS 1999). The British Thoracic Society (BTS) have advised that in patients with suspected PE, a leg ultrasound in those with coexisting clinical DVT is often sufficient as the initial imaging test to confirm VTE. However, a single leg ultrasound should not be relied upon for exclusion of subclinical DVT, so further testing may be required in asymptomatic patients (BTS 2003). As with most areas of practice, each patient needs an individual assessment. In patients with a low level of clinical suspicion for PE, a negative lung scan and a negative ultrasound of their legs, further testing is rarely merited. In a patient of high clinical suspicion and negative ultrasound and V/Q scan, the clinical likelihood of PE has been estimated at approximately 25%, and these patients generally go on to have angiography.

Pulmonary angiography

Historically considered the gold standard for diagnosis of PE, pulmonary angiography involves examination of the vasculature of the lungs by injecting radiocontrast material into the patient followed by fluoroscopy (direct X-ray visualization) of the lungs. PE is definitively diagnosed angiographically by the presence of an intraluminal filling defect in two views and demonstration of an occluded pulmonary artery. Secondary non-specific criteria include a reduction in perfusion and flow, tortuous peripheral vessels and delayed venous return (Newman 1989). The most common diagnostic algorithm for PE involves VQ scan followed by pulmonary angiography (typically CTPA).

Relative contraindications include significant bleeding risk and renal insufficiency. Patients with renal impairment must ensure that they are adequately hydrated before, during and after exposure to the contrast material. Complications of the procedure reported in large clinical trials include death (in five of 1111 patients; 0.5%), severe cardiopulmonary compromise (in four patients; 0.4%), renal failure requiring dialysis (three patients; 0.3%) and groin haematoma requiring blood transfusion (two patients; 0.2%) (ATS 1999).

Case study 6.1: a 'classic' case of cardiac chest pain

A 44 year-old overweight gentleman presented to the emergency department with a 4 hour history of central and right-sided chest pain. He described the pain as a dull ache which he first noticed on lying down in bed, with no radiation and nil difference with deep inspiration or coughing. The patient admitted to smoking 20 cigarettes a day and has been producing brown sputum, which is usual for him, but he did feel more short of breath than usual. There was no fever, nausea, vomiting, calf discomfort or other complaints. He was on no other medications and had an unremarkable past medical and family history. Examination reveals a slightly clammy obese patient with a heart rate of 103, a respiratory rate of 28 and

O₂ SATS (see Glossary) of 94% on air (note that he had received high-flow oxygen from the paramedic team *en route* to hospital). He was afebrile at 37 °C with a blood pressure of 135/93 and a BM of 7.6. Heart sounds were normal and chest examination revealed slightly decreased air entry bibasally but no focal crepitations or wheeze. On examination the patient had longstanding bilateral venous leg ulcers, which he had forgotten to mention, and no clinical evidence of DVT.

With regard to case study 6.1, which three investigations would you like to perform in the emergency department?

1. Electrocardiogram (ECG) – to rule out acute coronary syndrome (ACS), look for tachycardia and show any evidence of right heart strain.
2. Chest X-ray (CXR) – to look for any obvious consolidation/ effusions.
3. Arterial blood gas (ABG) – a more accurate assessment of the degree of hypoxia that O₂ SATS.

Start with simple accessible tests which help to rule in or rule out other diagnoses. It has been observed that the paradox in the diagnosis of PE is that it tends to be both under-diagnosed and over-investigated (Iles *et al.* 2003). First, always think of PE as a diagnosis and work through a mental list of patient risk factors combined with a pretest probability score. Second, when unsure, utilize the investigations above before proceeding to more invasive and expensive tests.

Arterial blood gas measurements taken on air:

- pH 7.432 (7.350–7.450).
- pCO₂ 4.45 (4.67–6.00).
- pO₂ 9.94 (10.00–13.33).
- ECG (see Figure 6.2).

Initial laboratory tests performed in the ED showed normal biochemistry and haemoglobin (Hb), with a slightly elevated white cell count (13.68). CXR showed a wedge-shaped opacity in the right mid-zone.

How will you decide if a D-dimer blood test is indicated in this patient?

A clinical pretest probability assessment should be made using a probability score such as the Geneva and Wells scores (see Tables 6.2 and

6.3). This patient would have a moderate probability for PE using the Geneva scoring system. The Wells criteria are more subjective. The patient scores 1.5 for being tachycardic, which in isolation would give him a low probability for PE; however, if you consider that PE is a more likely diagnosis than any other, which you could argue it is (there are no signs of infection and no signs of ischaemic changes on the ECG), then the patient gets three extra points and is now considered at moderate risk for PE. With a moderate probability assessment score the D-dimer is usually omitted, since further testing will be required regardless of the D-dimer result. In this particular case D dimer was taken on admission, along with the routine bloods, and was elevated at >1000.

Based on the history and examination, the patient is stable and has no features of a massive PE, so treatment in the ED is based on relief of symptoms with high-flow oxygen and analgesia and early administration of treatment-dose LMWH. Initial investigations are pointing towards a diagnosis of PE, but further confirmatory investigations are required. Many larger emergency departments now have 'PE protocols' in place (see Figure 6.1), which allow eligible patients to be investigated and managed in a clinical decisions unit and, if appropriate, started on oral anticoagulation on an outpatient basis. The patient in this case was admitted under the care of the medical team for CTPA and 12 hour measurement of cardiac enzymes, along with serial ECGs to exclude an acute coronary syndrome. CTPA confirmed PE and the patient was initiated on warfarin.

Treatment

Massive PE

Supportive treatment is key in the management of massive PE. Oxygen should be administered and patients may require analgesia. In hypotensive patients, plasma expanders and inotropic support may be required (see Box 6.2) (BTS 2003).

Thrombolysis

Thrombolytic therapy for PE remains controversial, due to the significant risk of major bleeding complications coupled with the increased costs (Arcasoy *et al.* 1999). Thrombolytics such as streptokinase, urokinase and recombinant tissue plasminogen activator (rt-PA; alteplase) directly dissolve intravascular thrombi by increasing plasmin levels (which breaks down fibrin and leads to clot lysis). This is different from

---

Box 6.2 Management of massive PE

Assess clinical state:

Cardiac arrest	Deteriorating	Stable condition
Resuscitation (CPR)	Contact consultant	80 U/kg i.v. heparin
50 mg i.v. alteplase	50 mg i.v. alteplase	Urgent echo or CTPA
Reassess at 30 minutes	Urgent echo or CTPA	

1. Massive PE likely if:
   - Collapse/hypotension and
   - Unexplained hypoxia and
   - Engorged neck veins and
   - Right ventricular gallop
2. In stable patients where massive PE is confirmed, i.v. dose of alteplase 100 mg in 90 minutes
3. Thrombolysis is followed by weight-adjusted UFH after 3 hours
4. Some units have facilities for clot fragmentation via pulmonary artery catheter if thrombolysis contraindicated. Elsewhere, contraindications to thrombolysis should be ignored in life-threatening PE.

(BTS 2003) reproduced with permission from the BMJ group

---

the action of anticoagulants, which prevent and reduce thrombus formation. Thrombolytics have several advantages over anticoagulation in the treatment of PE – they produce rapid clot lysis, resulting in faster improvements in pulmonary perfusion and gas exchange. They also eliminate the clot, which prevents recurrent PE and reduces the incidence of pulmonary hypertension from chronic vascular obstruction (Arcasoy et al. 1999).

The ACCP currently recommends the use of thrombolytic therapy in patients with evidence of haemodynamic compromise unless there are major contraindications to its use (see Box 6.3), although in the setting of massive PE causing shock, no contraindication is absolute (Arcasoy et al. 1999). It should be administered via a peripheral vein rather than by placing a pulmonary artery catheter, and short infusion times are recommended (Kearon et al. 2008). Thrombolytic therapy is more effective as soon after PE as possible, so treatment should not be delayed in appropriate patients (Kearon et al. 2008).

Box 6.3 Relative contraindications to thrombolytic therapy

- Recent (within 2 months) cerebrovascular accident, or intracranial or intraspinal trauma or surgery
- Active intracranial disease (aneurysm, vascular malformation, or neoplasm)
- Major internal bleeding within the past 6 months
- Uncontrolled hypertension (systolic BP >200 or diastolic BP 110 mmHg)
- Bleeding diathesis, including that associated with severe renal or hepatic disease
- Recent (within 10 days) major surgery, puncture of a non-compressible vessel, organ biopsy, or obstetric delivery
- Recent major and minor trauma, including cardiopulmonary resuscitation
- Infective endocarditis
- Pregnancy
- Haemorrhagic retinopathy
- Pericarditis
- Aneurysm

(Adapted from Arcasoy SM *et al.* 1999)

In patients with non-massive PE, use of thrombolysis is generally not recommended, since the risk of major haemorrhage is twice that with heparin (BTS 2003). Alteplase is the agent of choice in the United Kingdom, given as a 50 mg bolus (the same dose and route familiar to doctors treating myocardial infarction) (BTS 2003).

If thrombolysis fails, or there are contraindications, large emboli can be successfully fragmented using mechanical techniques, using a right heart catheter, or patients can have a surgical embolectomy. However, very few centres have these treatment options available to them (BTS 2003).

Vena caval filter

Placement of a IVC filter (Figure 6.5) is not carried out routinely but is indicated if patients have contraindications to anticoagulation, such as major bleeding, or if recurrent embolism is occurring despite being on adequate anticoagulant therapy (Kearon *et al.* 2008).

When faced with massive PE, when there is suspicion that additional emboli may be lethal and there are contraindications to thrombolytic therapy, filters are sometimes placed; however, this is not based

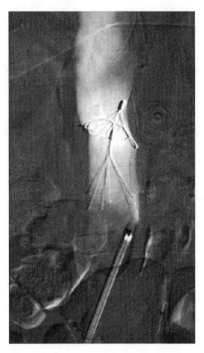

Figure 6.5 Inferior vena cava filter. A Simon Nitinol filter inserted in the vena cava of a pregnant women at high risk of VTE. Included with the permission of the King's Thrombosis Centre.

on firm trial data (Tapson 2008). They can be left in place permanently or retrieved several months later if no longer required. Recommendations for the use of vena cava filters have been published (Kaufman *et al.* 2006).

Anticoagulation

LMWH should be initiated as soon as PE is suspected, then, once reliably confirmed, oral anticoagulation should be commenced. A target INR of 2.0–3.0 is the aim and only once this has been achieved for more than 24 hours can heparin be discontinued (Kearon *et al.* 2008). Stable patients with PE can be considered as candidates for outpatient management (BTS 2003). Duration of therapy is three months for the first idiopathic episode and at least 6 months for other risk factors. The risk of bleeding should be balanced against the risk of further VTE. Anticoagulation for patients with VTE is outlined in the following chapter in more detail. For the BTS summary of the investigation and management of PE, please see Box 6.4.

Box 6.4 Summary of recommendations by the British Thoracic Society (BTS) for the investigation and management of PE

All patients with possible PE should have clinical probability assessed and an alternative clinical explanation should always be considered.

D-dimer

- D-dimer should only be carried out after clinical probability has been assessed and each hospital should provide information on the sensitivity and specificity of its D-dimer test.
- Those patients with a high clinical probability of PE should not have a D-dimer test performed.
- A negative D-dimer reliably excludes PE in those with low or intermediate clinical probability and such patients do not require further imaging.

Imaging

- CTPA is the initial lung imaging test of choice for non-massive PE.
- Patients with a good quality negative CTPA do not require further investigations or treatment for PE.
- Isotope lung scanning may be considered as the initial imaging investigation as long as imaging facilities are available on site, CXR is normal, there is no significant concurrent cardiopulmonary disease and standardized reporting criteria are used. A non-diagnostic result must always be followed by further imaging.
- Where isotope lung scanning is normal, PE is reliably excluded, but a significant minority of high-probability results are false positives.
- In patients with coexisting clinical DVT, lower limb ultrasound is often sufficient to confirm VTE; however. a single normal leg ultrasound should not be relied upon for exclusion of subclinical DVT.

Massive PE

- In the case of massive PE, CTPA will reliably confirm the diagnosis and thrombolysis is the first-line treatment; this may be initiated on clinical grounds alone if cardiac arrest is imminent (alteplase 50 mg bolus). Invasive management (thrombus fragmentation and IVC filter insertion) should be considered where facilities and expertise are available.

- Imaging should be performed within 1 hour in massive PE and ideally within 24 hours in non-massive PE.

Treatment

- Thrombolysis should not be first-line treatment in non-massive PE. Heparin should be given to intermediate and high-risk patients before imaging. LMWH is preferable, as it is easier to use, safer and has equal efficacy to UFH, but UFH can be considered as a first-dose bolus, in massive PE or where rapid reversal of effect may be needed.
- Oral anticoagulation should only be commenced once VTE is reliably confirmed. Target INR is 2.0–3.0; when this is achieved, heparin can be discontinued.
- The standard duration of oral anticoagulation is 4–6 weeks for patients with temporary risk factors, 3 months for first idiopathic and at least 6 months for other. Bleeding risk should be balanced with that of further VTE.
- Investigations for occult cancer are only indicated in idiopathic VTE when it is suspected clinically or on other routine tests. Testing for thrombophilia should be considered in patients under 50 with recurrent VTE or a strong family history of proven VTE.

(BTS 2003) reproduced with permission from the BMJ group

Case study 6.2: suddenly short of breath

A 70 year-old man is brought into the emergency department by the paramedics with new onset shortness of breath. He is alert and talking to you but vital signs show tachycardia (125 beats per minute), hypotension (80/50) and tachypnoea (35 breaths per minute). The doctor finds no abnormalities on the physical examination, but elicits from the history that the gentleman recently returned from a road trip to southern France and had been complaining of a painful right calf since then. ECG showed a sinus tachycardia and a RBBB. Chest X-ray showed a slightly enlarged right lung hilum but was otherwise unremarkable. D-dimers were sent, and were significantly elevated. Bedside transthoracic echocardiography (TTE) showed enlarged right heart chambers with moderate tricuspid regurgitation. The pulmonary artery was enlarged with evidence of thrombosis within the right pulmonary artery. Acute PE was diagnosed on the basis of these investigations.

What is the next step in the management of this patient?

In view of the patient's haemodynamic instability and the compelling evidence for a massive PE, thrombolysis should be administered. The patient has no contraindications to thrombolytic therapy and may die without clot lysis. Follow the protocol in place at your own place of work. BTS guidelines (2003) advise administration of 50mg i.v. alteplase, followed by an infusion of heparin. In an unstable patient, this can be given before investigations are carried out after discussion with a consultant – the earlier the better. Involve ICU early and consider inotropic support if the hypotension fails to improve.

What are the relative contraindications to thrombolytic therapy?

In life-threatening PE causing shock, no contraindication is absolute. The risk of bleeding is judged an acceptable risk to take if the alternative is death (Arcasoy *et al.* 1999). Relative contraindications are listed in Box 6.3 and include: recent cerebrovascular accident (within two months); intracranial or intraspinal trauma or surgery; active intracranial disease; major internal bleeding within the past six months; uncontrolled hypertension; bleeding diathesis; recent major surgery; puncture of a non-compressible vessel; organ biopsy or obstetric delivery within the preceding ten days; recent major and minor trauma, including cardiopulmonary resuscitation; infective endocarditis; pregnancy; haemorrhagic retinopathy; pericarditis; or an aneurysm (Arcasoy *et al.* 1999).

Case study 6.3: cardiac arrest

You are called to assist in the resuscitation of a 70 year-old gentleman who collapsed in the street. Passers-by found him unconscious and pulseless, so commenced cardiopulmonary resuscitation. Paramedics continued advanced life support en route to hospital and by the time the patient was wheeled into the emergency department he had a laryngeal mask airway *in situ* and had been shocked twice out of ventricular fibrillation, with a return of spontaneous circulation.

The patient is stabilized in the department and initial investigations carried out. Vitals show a blood pressure of 144/94, heart rate of 73 beats per minute, with sinus rhythm on the ECG, and SATS are 100% with the laryngeal mask airway (LMA) *in situ* and supplementary oxygen attached. Initial bloods are unremarkable and the chest X-ray is poor quality, but shows no obvious consolidation or pneumothorax. The patient's wife is present and tells you that he was in hospital a week ago with bleeding gastric ulcers and the doctors stopped his warfarin therapy, which he was taking for an irregular heart beat.

The ICU team are now involved and feel the patient is stable enough to have further investigations. The transthoracic echo demonstrates significant right ventricular dysfunction and the chest CT shows a pulmonary embolism in the distal left main pulmonary artery and also in the right descending pulmonary artery (a saddle embolism).

Why do you think the team have not proceeded straight to thrombolysis?

The patient has several relative contraindications to thombolysis, chiefly a recently gastric bleed and also recent cardiopulmonary resuscitation. It is a difficult decision, and depends upon the other treatment possibilities available at your institution. At present, the patient is stable, so there is time for the team to consider the options.

What other treatment options may be available for this patient with a saddle embolism?

The patient can have a surgical embolectomy or have the thrombus fragmented using mechanical techniques, followed by placement of an IVC filter to prevent recurrence in a patient who warfarin therapy is contraindicated. Indications for placement of an IVC include bleeding complications associated with anticoagulant therapy or any absolute contraindications to the use of anticoagulants. Patients who develop recurrent VTE despite adequate anticoagulation can also be considered as candidates. Filters aim to maintain caval patency, trap emboli, preserve prograde caval blood flow, avoid stasis and enhance the thrombolysis of trapped emboli.

Conclusion

The often vague, insidious symptoms of a PE mean that it is a condition that is often missed – with sometimes fatal consequences. After reading this chapter you should be aware of some of the different presentations of the condition and the signs and symptoms that should alert you to its presence. The use of clinical probability tools should be familiar to guide which investigations are used and you should be aware of the different management options available for massive and non-massive PE. The pharmacological management of VTE is discussed in the next chapter.

References

American Thoracic Society (ATS) (1999) The diagnostic approach to acute venous thromboembolism. Clinical practice guideline. *American Journal of Respiratory and Critical Care Medicine* **160**: 1043–1066.

Arcasoy SM, Kreit JW (1999) Thrombolytic therapy of pulmonary embolism. A comprehensive review of current evidence. *Chest* **115**: 1695–1707.

Bergqvist D, Lindblad B (1985) A 30 year survey of pulmonary embolisms verified at autopsy: an analysis of 1274 surgical patients. *British Journal of Surgery* **72**: 105–108.

Bastuji-Garin S, Schaeffer A, Wolkenstein P *et al.* (1998) Pulmonary embolism lung; scanning interpretation: about words. *Chest* **114**: 1551–1555.

British Nuclear Medicine Society (2003) Ventilation/perfusion imaging for pulmonary embolic disease. Available at: http://www.bnmsonline.co.uk/index.php?option=com_content&task=view&id=45&Itemid=151

British Thoracic Society (1997) Suspected acute pulmonary embolism-a practical approach. Thorax 52: (Suppl 3).

British Thoracic Society Standards of Care Committee Pulmonary Embolism Guideline Development Group (2003) British Thoracic Society guidelines for the management of suspected acute pulmonary embolism. *Thorax* **58**: 470–484.

Burkill GJ, Bell JR, Padley SP (1999) Survey on the use of pulmonary scintigraphy; spiral CT and conventional pulmonary angiography for suspected pulmonary embolism in the British Isles. *Clinical Radiology* **54**: 807–810.

Courtney DM, Sasser H, Pincus B *et al.* (2001) Pulseless electrical activity with witnessed arrest as a predictor of sudden death from massive pulmonary embolism in outpatients. *Resuscitation* **49**: 265–273.

Dieter RS, Ernst E, Ende DJ *et al.* (2002) Diagnostic utility of cardiac troponin-I levels in patients with suspected pulmonary embolism. *Angiology* **53**: 583–585.

Dorfman GS, Cronan JJ, Tupper TB *et al.* (1987) Occult pulmonary embolism: a common occurrence in deep venous thrombosis. *American Journal of Radiology* **148**: 263–266.

Douketis JD (2002) Elevated cardiac troponin levels in patients with submassive pulmonary embolism. *Archives of Internal Medicine* **162**: 79–81.

Fiappo E, Quattrin R, Calligaris L *et al.* (2009) Appropriate laboratory utilisation in diagnosing pulmonary embolism. *Annals of Clinical Biochemistry* **46**: 18–23.

Forbes KP, Reid JH, Murchison JT (2001) Do preliminary chest X-ray findings define the optimum role of pulmonary scintigraphy in suspected pulmonary embolism? *Clinical Radiology* **56**: 397–400.

Giannitsis E, Muller-Bardorff M, Kurowski V *et al.* (2000) Independent prognostic value of cardiac troponin in patients with confirmed pulmonary embolism. *Circulation* **102**: 211–217.

Goldhaber SZ, Hennekens CH, Evans DA *et al.* (1982) Factors associated with correct antemortem diagnosis of major pulmonary embolism. *American Journal of Medicine* **73**: 822–826.

Green RM, Meyer TJ, Dunn M, Glassroth J (1992) Pulmonary embolism in younger adults. *Chest* **101**: 1507–1511.

Hartmann I, Hagen P, Melissant C *et al.* (2000) Diagnosing acute pulmonary embolism: effect of chronic obstructive pulmonary disease on the performance of D-dimer testing, ventilation/perfusion scintigraphy, spiral computed tomographic angiography and concentional angiography. *American Journal of Respiratory and Critical Care Medicine* **162**: 2232–2237.

Hull RD, Hirsh J, Carter CJ *et al.* (1983) Pulmonary angiography, ventilation lung scanning and venography for clinically suspected pulmonary embolism with abnormal lung perfusion scan. *Annals of Internal Medicine* **98**: 891–899.

Iles S, Beckert L, Than M *et al.* (2003) Making a diagnosis of pulmonary embolism new methods and clinical issues. *New Zealand Journal of Medicine* **116**: 1177.

Iwadate K, Tanno K, Doi M *et al.* (2001) Two cases of right ventricular ischemic injury due to massive pulmonary embolism. *Forensic Science International* **116**: 189–195.

Janata K, Holzer M, Laggner AN *et al.* (2003) Cardiac troponin T in the severity assessment of patients with pulmonary embolism: cohort study. *British Medical Journal* **326**: 312–313.

Kasper W, Konstantinides S, Geibel A *et al.* (1997) Prognostic significance of right ventricular afterload stress detected by echocardiography in patients with clinically suspected pulmonary embolism. *Heart* **77**: 346–349.

Kaufman JA, Kinney TB, Streiff ME *et al.* (2006) Guidelines for the use of retrievable and convertible vena cava filters: report from the Society of Interventional Radiology multidisciplinary consensus conference. *Journal of Vascular Interventional Radiology* **17**: 449–459.

Kearon C, Kahn S, Agnelli G *et al.* (2008) Antithrombotic therapy for venous thromboembolic disease: ACCP evidence based clinical practice guidelines, 8th Edition. *Chest* **133**: 454–545.

Lindblad B, Erkson A, Bergquist D (1991) Autopsy verified pulmonary embolism in a surgical department: analysis of the period from 1951 to 1988. *British Journal of Surgery* **78**: 849–852.

McNeill BJ, Hessel SJ, Branch WT *et al.* (1976) Measures of clinical efficacy: the value of the lung scan in the evaluation of young patients with pleuritic chest pain. *Journal of Nuclear Medicine* **17**: 163–164.

McNeil BJ (1976) A diagnostic strategy using ventilation-perfusion studies in patients suspect for pulmonary embolism. *Journal of Nuclear Medicine* **17**: 613–616.

Monreal M, Ruiz J, Olazabal A *et al.* (1992) Deep venous thrombosis and the risk of pulmonary embolism. *Chest* **102**: 677–681.

Newman GE, Sullivan DC, Gottschalk A *et al.* (1972) Scintigraphic perfusion patterns in patients with diffuse lung disease. *Radiology* **143**: 227–231.

Newman GE (1989) Pulmonary angiography in pulmonary embolism. *Journal of Thoracic Imaging* **4**: 28–39.

Nilsson T, Mare K, Carlsson A (2001) Value of structured clinical and scintigraphic protocols in acute pulmonary embolism. *Journal of Internal Medicine* **250**: 213–218.

Pineda LA, Hathwar VS, Grant BJB (2001) Clinical suspicion of fatal pulmonary embolism. *Chest* **120**: 791–796.

PIOPED Investigators (1990) Value of the ventilation-perfusion scan in acute pulmonary embolism: results of the Prospective Investigation of Pulmonary Embolism Diagnosis (PIOPED). *Journal of the American Medical Association* **263**: 2753–2759.

Prologo JD, Glauser J (2002) Variable diagnostic approach to suspected pulmonary embolism in the ED of a major academic tertiary care center. *American Journal of Emergency Medicine* **20**: 5–9.

Righini M, Goehring C, Bounameaux H *et al.* (2000) Effects of age on the performance of common diagnostic tests for pulmonary embolism. *American Journal of Medicine* **109**: 357–361.

Robinson GV (2006) Pulmonary embolism in hospital practice. *British Medical Journal* **332**: 156–160.

Saeger W, Genzkow M (1994) Venous thromboses and pulmonary embolisms in post mortem series: probable causes by correlations of clinical data and basic diseases. *Pathology Research and Practise* **190**: 394–399.

Sharma S (2006) Pulmonary embolism. Emedicine. Available at: http://emedicine.medscape.com/article/300901-diagnosis

Sokolove PE, Offerman SR (2001) Pulmonary embolism. *New England Journal of Medicine* **345**: 1311.

Stein PD, Gottschalk A (1974) Critical review of ventilation-perfusion lung scans in acute pulmonary embolism. *Progress in Cardiovascular Diseases* **37**: 13–24.

Stein PD, Terrin ML, Hales CA *et al.* (1991) Clinical, laboratory, roentgeno-graphic and electrocardiographic findings in patients with acute pulmonary embolism and no pre-existing cardiac or pulmonary disease. *Chest* **100**: 598–603.

Tapson VF (2008) Acute pulmonary embolism. *New England Journal of Medicine* **358**: 1037–1052.

Anonymous (1973) Urokinase Pulmonary Embolism Trial: a national co-operative study. *Circulation* **47**(Suppl II): 1–108.

Van Beek EJR, Brouwers EMJ, Song B *et al.* (2001) Lung scintigraphy and helical computed tomography for the diagnosis of pulmonary embolism: a meta-analysis. *Clinical and Applied Thrombosis and Hemostasis* **7**: 87–92.

Velchik MG, Tobin M, McCarthy K (1989) Nonthromboembolic causes of high probability lung scans. *American Journal of Physiologic Imaging* **4**: 32–38.

Wells PS, Anderson DR, Rodger M *et al.* (2000) Derivation of a simple clinical model to categorize patients probability of pulmonary embolism: Increasing the models Utility with the SimpliRED d-dimer. *Thrombosis and Haemostasis* **83**(3): 416–420.

Wicki J, Pemeger TV, Junod AF *et al.* (2001) Assessing clinical probability of pulmonary embolism in the emergency ward: a simple score. *Archives of Internal Medicine* **161**: 92–97.

Pharmacological management of VTE

Overview

The pharmacological management of VTE is outlined in detail in this chapter. The three major classes of anticoagulants currently licensed for use for VTE in the United Kingdom are examined individually, covering their pharmacokinetics, indications and contraindications. Initiation of therapy and intensity and duration of treatment is covered and the need for monitoring is explained. The main adverse effect of anticoagulation is bleeding, and pointers are given on how to manage bleeding patients taking anticoagulants. The drugs and dietary interactions known to increase bleeding risk are outlined and the use of anticoagulants in specific high-risk groups is discussed.

Introduction

Antithrombotic therapy is used for numerous arterial and venous thromboembolic conditions to help prevent occlusive vascular disease in patients at risk of thrombosis. Antithrombotic agents are classified by their mechanism of action. Anticoagulants block the production and

Venous Thromboembolism: A Nurses Guide to Prevention and Management   By Ellen Welch
© 2010 John Wiley & Sons, Ltd.

activation of the clotting factors. Antiplatelet agents interfere with platelet activation or aggregation. Fibrinolytics enzymatically dissolve the fibrin component of thrombin. Their different modes of action mean that they have different indications and contraindications.

There are three classes of anticoagulants currently licensed for VTE in the United Kingdom:

- Vitamin K antagonists (VKAs), such as warfarin.
- Heparins, which include unfractionated heparin (UFH), low molecular weight heparin (LMWH) and synthetic pentasaccharides (factor Xa inhibitors) such as fondaparinux.
- Direct thrombin inhibitors (DTIs).

Vitamin K antagonists (VKAs)

Vitamin K antagonists, such as warfarin and other coumarin anticoagulants, have been available for more than 50 years (see Box 7.1). These drugs are commonly referred to as 'oral anticoagulants'; however, the term 'vitamin K antagonists' (VKAs) is preferred, as it helps to distinguish them from other agents that are currently being developed (and will be discussed later), such as oral inhibitors of activated factor X and oral thrombin inhibitors (Schulman 2003). Since warfarin is the most commonly used VKA, and has more data available relevant to its use, the terms 'warfarin' and 'VKA' are used interchangeably.

VKAs are 'blood thinners', not 'clot busters'. They have no direct effect on an established thrombus and they cannot reverse the ischaemic tissue damage brought about by a clot. They therefore do not 'treat' VTE. The aim of anticoagulation therapy is to prevent further clot progression and secondary thromboembolic complications (Baker et al. 2004). They act by lowering the amount of active vitamin K available for the activation of the vitamin K-dependent coagulation factors II, VII, IX and X – their mechanism of action is discussed further in Chapter 2 (Box 2.4, p. 33). The major concern with the use of anticoagulant therapy is the risk of bleeding complications. The annual incidence of major haemorrhage (defined as intracranial haemorrhage or bleeding necessitating transfusion or hospitalization) was found to be in the range 1.2–7 episodes per 100 patients in different cohort studies, whereas the incidence of minor bleeding was reported as 2–24 episodes per 100 patients (Schulman 2001).

Long-term anticoagulation must therefore be initiated with care, and each individual patient should be assessed for predictors of haemorrhagic complications and consideration given to the duration and

---

Box 7.1 The discovery of warfarin

In 1922, a haemorrhagic disease was described in cattle, which was linked to mouldy sweet clover hay. Sweet clover provided a nutritious meal for livestock when fresh or as hay, but if the hay became spoiled, cattle were noted to develop severe spontaneous bleeding (Schofield 1922). It was observed that the affected cattle had a diminished quantity of the clotting factor prothrombin, and subsequent research led to the isolation and purification of the responsible 'haemorrhagic agent' in the spoiled sweet clover, dicumarol (3,3-methylene-bis-[4-hydroxycoumarin]) (Overman *et al.* 1941). Dicumarol is derived from the oxidation of coumarin (the plant product responsible for the distinctive sweet smell of clover) by the action of fungi in the mouldy hay (Scully 2002).

Warfarin was discovered in 1946 and was initially launched as the ideal rat poison. Dicumarol proved to be ineffective as a rodenticide, but its derivative, 3-phenylacetyl ethyl 4-hydroxycoumarin, otherwise known as warfarin, was much more potent. Its name is an acronym for the research institution where it was synthesized – the Wisconsin Alumni Research Foundation. Warfarin was initially considered too toxic for use in humans, but in 1951 a failed suicide attempt by a navy recruit, who took a large dose of rat poison, led clinicians to discard dicumarol in favour of warfarin. In 1999 warfarin was the eleventh most prescribed drug in the USA, with annual sales of approximately US$500 million (Scully 2002).

---

intensity of therapy, with adequate monitoring and education provided. VKAs are contraindicated in peptic ulcer disease, severe hypertension, bacterial endocarditis and pregnancy [*British National Formulary* (BNF) 2008].

Pharmacokinetics

Warfarin is highly water-soluble and is rapidly absorbed after oral administration, reaching peak concentrations in plasma within 60–90 minutes (Schulman 2001). Once in the circulation, 98–99% of warfarin is bound to albumin, therefore only a fraction is biologically active. The elimination half-life in in the range 35–45 hours and the duration of effect is 2–5 days (Baker *et al.* 2004). Warfarin is eliminated almost entirely by metabolism, mainly in the liver, with very little excreted unchanged in the urine and bile. The other VKAs currently used therapeutically as anticoagulants do not differ in their effect on vitamin K metabolism, but they have differences in elimination. The elimination half-life of acenocoumarol is 3–10 hours and that of phenprocoumon is 90–140 hours, which has management implications. Phenprocoumon takes over two weeks to reach a steady state, whereas acenocoumarol has to be administered twice daily (Scully 2002).

Indications

VTE is not the only condition in which VKAs are used. Patients with valvular heart disease (i.e. rheumatic mitral valve disease, mitral valve prolapse, mitral regurgitation, mitral annular calcification or mobile aortic atheromas) are at risk of systemic embolization and benefit from therapy (Stein *et al.* 2001). Warfarin is used to reduce the incidence of ischaemic stroke in patients with atrial fibrillation (Albers *et al.* 2001). It also has proven efficacy in the treatment of coronary artery disease (Cairns *et al.* 2001). Controversial indications are peripheral arterial disease, heart failure and dissecting carotid artery aneurysm (Schulman 2003). The suggested target INRs for these conditions are shown in Table 7.1. For further information on these conditions, please refer to a more detailed text.

Initiation

Patients with VTE should be anticoagulated as soon as the diagnosis is confirmed. Warfarin inhibits protein C and protein S along with other vitamin K-dependent coagulation factors, as explained in Chapter 2. This creates an initially hypercoagulable state (i.e. an increased tendency towards blood clotting), which is why initial treatment of VTE

Table 7.1 Indications and target INRs

Indication	Target INR
Prevention of systemic embolism	
Mechanical prosthetic heart valves	2.5–3.5
Bioprosthetic heart valves	2.0–3.0
Non-valvular atrial fibrillation	2.0–3.0
Myocardial infarction	2.0–3.0
Mitral valve disease in sinus rhythm	2.0–3.0
Prevention of recurrent disease	
Ischaemic stroke in atrial fibrillation	2.0–3.0
Myocardial infarction	2.0–3.0
Venous thromboembolism	2.0–3.0

(Adapted from Schulman 2003; Hirsh *et al.* 2001)

involves using both heparin and warfarin together. A randomized controlled study showed that there was a threefold increase in recurrent VTE in patients treated with VKAs alone compared with VKAs combined with heparin therapy (Brandjes *et al.* 1992).

In the past, the initiation of the VKA was delayed, but current advice is to start heparin and a VKA together on day 1 of treatment (Kearon *et al.* 2008). Simultaneous introduction of the two agents has not been found to lead to more recurrences or haemorrhages than does delaying the initiation of VKA, and it reduces the duration of heparin treatment, which decreases the risk of heparin-induced thrombocytopenia (Schulman 2003). Heparin treatment should be continued for at least 5 days until the INR is >2.0 for 24 hours (Kearon *et al.* 2008).

The large 'loading doses' of VKAs that were previously used when initiating therapy have been abandoned, since they frequently caused haemorrhage (Schulman 2001). Warfarin is generally initiated at a dose of 2.5–10 mg, although the variability in dose requirements is wide (Kearon *et al.* 2008). Dosing variability is thought to be due to differences in clearance of the drug by the liver. Observational studies have shown that lower VKA maintenance doses are required in older patients, women and those with impaired nutrition and vitamin K deficiency (Kearon *et al.* 2008). A dose of 10 mg is suggested in younger (i.e. <60 years) and otherwise healthy outpatients. Older patients, those that are hospitalized and those at a higher risk of bleeding are recommended to start at a dose of 5 mg (Kearon *et al.* 2008).

Main pointers in the initiation of therapy are (Baker *et al.* 2004):

- Avoid high loading doses of warfarin, which may precipitate bleeding.
- Consider potential drug interactions.
- Aim for an INR that balances the therapeutic goal with the risk factors for bleeding on an individual basis.
- A reduced target INR range has not been proved to reduce bleeding risk and can lead to ineffective therapy.
- Avoid frequent dose adjustments. Remember, a dose change will take several days to influence INR.
- Avoid excessive increases in doses when the INR drifts below the target range.
- Ensure effective patient education.

Intensity of treatment

The daily maintenance dose of warfarin varies greatly between individual patients, from 0.5 to 15 mg per day, and often fluctuates over time (Gallus *et al.* 2000). INR is measured daily or on every second day during initiation of therapy, with the dose of warfarin titrated against the INR (see section on Monitoring, below). Table 7.1 outlines the range of target INR values for different conditions at which the incidence of thromboembolism and major haemorrhage are both lowest. The target INR in patients with VTE is 2.5 (range 2.0–3.0).

The risk of progression or recurrence of VTE decreases with time as the thrombus resolves or is covered over by endothelium and the activation of coagulation therefore subsides, in patients with unprovoked DVT who have a strong preference for less frequent INR testing to monitor their therapy, after the first three months of conventional intensity anticoagulation (i.e. range 2.0–3.0). The American College of Chest Physicians (ACCP) recommend low-intensity therapy (INR range, 1.5–1.9) with less frequent monitoring, rather than stopping treatment completely (Kearon *et al.* 2008; Schulman 2003). High-intensity therapy (INR range 3.0–4.5) has been shown to be associated with high rates of bleeding in patients with VTE (Hull *et al.* 1982).

Duration of treatment

Anticoagulant therapy for VTE should be continued until either the benefits (reduction of recurrent VTE) no longer clearly outweigh its risks of bleeding or, alternatively, the patient wishes to stop the treatment (Kearon *et al.* 2008).

The risk of recurrent VTE is influenced by the location and extension of the thrombus, by the nature of the risk factors and whether they are permanent or reversible, and by resolution of the acute episode of VTE (Schulman 2003; Kearon *et al.* 2008). Warfarin is usually given for 3–6 months after VTE. Controversies exist regarding the optimal duration of treatment and many studies suggest that it should be determined by the patient's clinical presentation. For example, in patients with reversible risk factors (such as transient immobilization postoperatively) with symptomatic calf vein DVT (which is considered clinically unimportant), 6–12 weeks of warfarin therapy is thought to be sufficient (Van der Meer *et al.* 1993), while patients with idiopathic episodes where there is a continuing cause, such as cancer or an inherited or acquired 'hypercoaguable state', may require therapy for longer than 6 months (Gallus *et al.* 2000).

The current recommendations compiled by the ACCP are outlined in Table 7.2.

There are many disadvantages to the patient's quality of life while taking warfarin, such as the need for frequent venepuncture, the numerous drug interactions and the complex adjustments needed for

Table 7.2 ACCP recommendations – duration of anticoagulant therapy for VTE

Type of event	Duration of VKA therapy
VTE secondary to a transient (reversible) risk factor	3 months
Unprovoked VTE	3 months then risk/benefits evaluated regarding long-term therapy
Second episode of unprovoked VTE	Long-term treatment
VTE and cancer	Long-term treatment (or until cancer resolves). LMWH recommended for first 3–6 months

patients undergoing surgical procedures. In patients receiving long-term anticoagulant therapy, the risk : benefit ratio should be reassessed at periodic intervals – at least annually.

Discontinuing therapy may be carried out either abruptly or gradually, since no difference in the risk of clinical events between the two approaches has been identified (Ascani *et al.* 1999).

Monitoring

In the laboratory
Anticoagulation therapy is monitored by measuring the prothrombin time (PT). The PT responds to a reduction by of three of the four vitamin K-dependent clotting factors (II, VII and X), reflecting the activity of the extrinsic and common pathways of the coagulation cascade (see Chapter 2, Box 2.3, p. 28).

The PT assay is carried out in the laboratory by adding a thromboplastin extract of a tissue (usually lung, brain or placenta containing the tissue factor and phospholipid necessary to promote the activation of factor X by factor VII) to citrated plasma, which is then recalcified to initiate the reaction (Hirsh *et al.* 2001; Schulman 2001).

In the 1980s it was noted that there is a wide variety in the sensitivities of the thromboplastins used between different laboratories, depending on their source, phospholipid content and preparation, which made multicentre comparisons of treatment impossible to interpret. This led to the development of the International Normalised Ratio (INR) to standardize the reporting of PT between different centres (Loeliger *et al.* 1985). The INR is a calibration system which allows different laboratories to adjust the PT ratios obtained using their local reagents and instruments, to enable comparison with the universal standard. The formula is based on a linear relationship between the logarithms of PT ratios obtained with the reference and test thromboplastins:

$$INR = (PT_{patient}/PT_{control})ISI$$

where the International Sensitivity Index (ISI) is a correction factor for the responsiveness of the thromboplastin to the reductions in the vitamin K-dependent coagulation factors (Schulman 2001). An unresponsive thromboplastin produces less prolongation of the PT for a given reduction in vitamin K-dependent clotting factors than a responsive thromboplastin. The lower the ISI, the more responsive the reagent (Hirsh *et al.* 2001). Simply put, the INR is the PT ratio that would be obtained if every sample was analysed using the same controlled assay.

Frequency

In patients starting a VKA, INR monitoring should be started after the initial two or three doses have been taken and then carried out every day or every other day. INR is then measured less frequently, depending on the response of the patient. An INR within 0.5 units of the target value is generally satisfactory; larger deviations require dosing adjustment. Once a steady state is reached, most patients receiving a stable dose of oral anticoagulants remain well controlled with 4–6 weekly testing and dose adjustment, while others need more frequent assessment (Gallus *et al.* 2000; Kearon *et al.* 2008).

During the first few days of VKA therapy, the prolonged PT (increased INR) reflects the clearance of coagulation factor VII. This initial elevation is not thought to be associated with a clinically important antithrombotic effect. It is the later reduction of coagulation factors II and X which exerts the major antithrombotic effect, which occurs much more slowly (72–90 hours) (Hirsh *et al.* 2001; Schulman 2001). As already mentioned, warfarin blocks synthesis of the functional vitamin K-dependent coagulation factors (II, VII, IX, X, protein C, protein S). However, its impact on the INR is delayed until the coagulation factors already formed before warfarin was administered are removed (Gallus *et al.* 2000). Because of this, the maximum effect of a dose occurs up to 48 hours after initial administration, with the effects lasting for the next five days (Baker *et al.* 2004).

Various computer programs, nomograms and flexible protocols have been developed to improve the selection of initial and maintenance dosing of VKA (Poller *et al.* 1998). Portable instruments suitable for home use have also been developed which, with the appropriate training, allow patients to monitor their own INR and make dosing adjustments (Anderson *et al.* 1993). These tools have improved outcomes for patients by reducing the number of dose adjustments needed, shortening the time to achieve steady state and reducing the number of INR values outside the therapeutic range (Ageno *et al.* 1998). Such resources allow non-physicians to make dose adjustments, allowing anticoagulation to be achieved in a larger variety of clinical settings. Whoever is managing the anticoagulation therapy needs to take a systematic approach, incorporating regular INR testing, follow-up and effective communication of results and dosing decisions. With appropriate education and help from supportive tools, motivated patients can be taught to monitor the PT and adjust their own doses themselves (Schulman 2003). In patients who are suitably selected and trained, self-testing and self-management has been found to be effective (Kearon *et al.* 2008).

Anticoagulant therapy is often suboptimal in routine practice, with a high proportion of INR results outside of the target range (Pell *et al.* 1993). The reason for unstable INRs may be problems with reagents and instruments in the laboratory, staff and patient factors, and largely due to the many interactions VKAs have with a number of substances, as outlined below.

Drug interactions

To achieve safe anticoagulation, it is important that both the patient and healthcare provider are aware of the important interactions VKAs can have with other drugs and foods. The list of drugs that interact with warfarin and other VKAs is extensive (see Boxes 7.2 and 7.3) and ever-expanding, and any change to a patient's medication should involve making reference to the *British National Formulary* or a drug reference book to ensure that you are aware of possible interactions.

It can take several days for the effects of changes to take place, so an INR measured approximately 1 one week after a change in medication should reflect significant interactions (Baker *et al.* 2004). There are many case reports in the literature of interactions with warfarin; however, a recent paper suggests that many of these are of poor quality and present potentially misleading conclusions about drug use (Holbrook *et al.* 2005). Case reports represent the 'lowest level' in the hierarchy of evidence, with no standardization to their presentation – meaning that the quality can be variable. However, they still serve a useful purpose and provide a reminder that interactions can occur.

The most consistent reports of interactions are with drugs that can influence either the absorption or metabolic clearance of warfarin, including azole antibiotics, macrolides, quinolones, non-steroidal anti-inflammatory drugs, selective serotonin reuptake inhibitors,

Box 7.2 Drug interactions with warfarin and other vitamin K antagonists (causing an *increased* anticoagulant response)

Acarbose
ACETAMINOPHEN/PARACETAMOL
Allopurinol
Aminoglycosdies
Aminosaliclic acid
AMIODARONE
Amoxicillin
ANDROGENS
Azapropazone
Azathioprine
Azithromycin
Benzbromarone
Benziodarone
β-Adrenergic blockers
Bezafibrate
Bromodeoxyuridine
Carboplatin
Cefamandole
Chloral hydrate
Chloramphenicol
CIMETIDINE
Ciprofloxacin
Citalopram
Clarithromycin
CLOFIBRATE
Corticosteroids (high-dose)
Danazole
Defoperazone
Dextropropoxyphene
Diazoxide
Diflunisal
Disopyramide
DISULFIRAM
ERYTHROMYCIN
Ethacrinic acid
Etoposide
Felbamate
Feprazone

Flubiprophen
FLUCONAZOLE
5-Fluorouracil
FLUOXETINE
Flutamide
Fluvastatin
Fluvoxamine
Gemfibrozil
GLUCAGON
Halofenate
Hydrocodone
Indomethacin
Influenze vaccine
Interferon
Isoniazid
Isoxicam
Itraconazole
Ketoconazole
Ketoprophen
Levamisole
Lovastatin
Meclofenamate
Mefenamic acid
Mesna
Methylsalicylate
METRONIDAZOLE
Miconazole
Moricizine
Moxolactam
Nalidixic acid
Norfloxacin
Ofloxacin
Omeprazole
OXYPHENBUTAZONE
Paroxetine
PHENYLBUTAZONE
Phenyramidol
Phenytoin

Piroxicam
Pravastatin
Propafenone
Propoxyphene
Propranolol
Quinidine
Ranitidine
SALICYLATES (HIGH-DOSE)
Saquinavir
Sertralin
Simvastatin
SULFAMETHOXAZOLE–
  TRIMETHOPRIM
SULFINPYRAZONE
Sulfonamides
Sulindac

TAMOXIFEN
Tenidap
Terbinafine
Tetracyclines
THYROID
HORMONE
Tiaprofenoic acid
Tolmentin
Toremiphen
Tramadol
Tricyclic
antidepressants
Vitamin E
Zileuton
Zolpidem

Drugs with profound or frequent interactions appear in CAPITALS.
(Data extracted from Schulman 2001; also check *British National Formulary*)

Box 7.3 Drug interactions with warfarin and other vitamin K antagonists (causing a *decreased* anticoagulant response)

Aminoglutethimide
Antipyrine
ANTITHYROID DRUGS
Ascorbic acid
Azathioprine
BARBITURATES
CARBAMAZAPINE
CHOLESTYRAMINE
Contraceptives, oral
Cyclophosphamide
DICHLORALPHENAZONE
Dicloxacillin
Ethchlorvynol
Etretinate
Flucloxacillin
Furosemide
Glucocorticoids

GLUTETHIMIDE
Griseofulvin
Mercaptopurine
Methaqualone
Mianserine
Mitotane
Nafcillin
Propofol
Rifampicin
Simethicone
Spironolactone
Sucralfate
Teicoplanin
Thiazide diuretics
Trazodone
Ubidecarone

Drugs with profound or frequent interactions appear in CAPITALS.
(Data extracted from Schulman 2001; also check *British National Formulary*)

omeprazole, amiodarone, lipid-lowering agents and fluorouracil. Co-administration of these medications with warfarin should be either avoided or closely monitored (Holbrook *et al.* 2005).

Elderly patients often exhibit an exaggerated response to warfarin, thought to be due to their depleted stores of vitamin K (Hirsh *et al.* 2001). Incidentally, the effects of VKAs have reportedly been increased during the summer months, which has been linked to exposure to insecticides such as ivermectin or metidation (Fernandez *et al.* 1998).

High risk drugs

The most difficult drugs to manage when combined with warfarin are those that can cause bleeding on their own, such as other anticoagulants (heparin), antiplatelet drugs (acetylsalicylic acid, clopidogrel, dipyridamole) and all non-steroidal anti-inflammatory drugs (NSAIDs), including the COX2-selective NSAIDs. All of these drugs should generally be avoided in combination with warfarin, unless proven to provide benefit that outweighs the risks (Holbrook *et al.* 2005).

Alternative medicines

The use of alternative medicines and supplements, such as vitamins, minerals, amino acids, herbal and other natural products, is on the increase (Eisenberg *et al.* 1998). However, patients are rarely made aware of possible interactions with these substances, which are readily available over the counter. A study from the United States showed that 61% of outpatients with cardiovascular disease taking supplements did not have any information about the risks, benefits and adverse effects of their alternative medication or about potential interactions with prescription drugs (Wood *et al.* 2003).

Among 1203 patients taking warfarin, a study showed that 31% regularly took one or more dietary supplements, most commonly glucosamine, fish oil, cranberry extract, green tea, coenzyme Q10 and grapefruit extract, all of which have been reported to interact with warfarin (Wittkowsky *et al.* 2007).

To ensure patient safety, it is suggested that all herbal supplements be avoided in patients taking warfarin, due to the lack of quality control regarding their contents (Holbrook *et al.* 2005). Practically, however, patients do not want to be denied the choice to use supplements, especially when the risks are largely anecdotal. Patients should be educated on possible interactions with warfarin and herbal medications, and physicians should remember to specifically ask about their use. Table 7.3 lists herbal supplements and foods that have been shown to have clinically significant interactions with warfarin. Most of the interactions

Table 7.3 Herbal supplements and foods that interact with warfarin

Potentiate the effect	Inhibit the effect
Fish oil	High vitamin K content foods
Mango	Avocado
Boldo-fenugreek	Soy milk
Quilinggao	Ginseng
Grapefruit juice	Sushi containing seaweed
Danshen	Green tea
Dong quai	
Lycium barbarum L	
PC-SPES	
Cranberry juice	

(Adapted from Holbrook et al. 2005)

reported have no documented mechanism. Green tea contains vitamin K and therefore antagonizes warfarin. Commonly used supplements such as St John's wort, ginseng and garlic may lower the concentration of warfarin in the blood, while ginkgo is associated with bleeding when taken with warfarin (Izzo et al. 2001).

A registry of interactions between dietary supplements and anticoagulants is currently being developed through Clotcare Online Resource (http://www.clotcare.com). It was recognized that there is a paucity of information surrounding the impact of dietary supplements in patients taking warfarin (Bussey et al. 2005). This database aims to remedy this by enabling the collection of high quality case-based evidence of interactions that occur in stable anticoagulated patients (Wittkowsky 2008).

In the United Kingdom, detection and recording of any adverse drug reactions or interactions is carried using the 'Yellow Card' scheme. Suspected adverse reactions to any therapeutic agent should be reported to: www.yellowcard.gov.uk

Dietary interactions

The amount of vitamin K in the diet can determine the effect of treatment with VKAs. Vitamin K1 (phylloquinone) is the main form present in our diets and is found mainly in dark green vegetables, such as spinach and broccoli. Detailed advice regarding diet should be given to patients to avoid the common response adopted by many patients, which is to omit vegetables from their diet completely. Very few reactions between VKAs and food are clinically relevant. Studies have

---

Box 7.4 A balanced diet during warfarin therapy

- Be consistent. Avoid major changes to your diet. If change is necessary, talk to your doctor and arrange to temporarily increase the frequency of monitoring.
- Avoid avocado, kale, parsley and the Japanese dish natto, except as a garnish/minor ingredient.
- Choose up to one serving of green vegetables (100 g) per day (e.g. broccoli, brussels sprouts, spinach).
- Discuss with your doctor any increased or decreased intake of vitamin K-rich foods (e.g. lentils, garbanzo beans, soybeans, soybean oil, liver, green tea).
- Alcohol intake should be discouraged.
- Vitamin E supplements appear to interact with vitamin K, so should be avoided.
- Vitamin A and C supplements have occasionally caused changes in prothrombin time, therefore doses higher than the recommended daily allowance should be avoided.
- In patients with poorly controlled anticoagulation in which no obvious reason can be identified, a diet with a consistent vitamin K content may be beneficial.

(Adapted from Schulman 2001)

---

shown that large amounts of broccoli can cause warfarin resistance (Kempin 1983) and that a large intake of avocado oils seem to also antagonize warfarin (Blickstein *et al.* 1991). However, quite substantial amounts are needed to cause an effect. Prothrombin time is not effected by 250 g broccoli or spinach eaten on a single occasion, but larger portions than this do start to show an effect (Karlson *et al.* 1986). Rather than restricting vegetable intake, it is better to recommend a consistent, balanced diet, as outlined in Box 7.4, and to be aware of potential problems during situations of dietary change, such as illness, travel, fad diets, hospitalization and during the postoperative period (Baker *et al.* 2004).

Beverages

Alcohol in moderation has little effect on the metabolism of warfarin; however, in heavy drinkers factors such as alcohol-induced gastritis, poor diet, increased falls and poor compliance all increase the risk of bleeding (Campbell *et al.* 2001). Any significant changes to alcohol consumption, such as binge drinking, should be avoided, and a limit of two alcoholic drinks per day is suggested (Tatsumi *et al.* 2007).

There has been much debate over the safety of drinking common beverages such as cranberry juice and grapefruit juice while taking certain medications. Grapefruit juice has been shown to augment plasma levels and therefore increase the effects of several medications (e.g. statins). Natural substances present in grapefruit juice (primarily furanocoumarin derivatives) have the capacity to inhibit enzymes in the gastrointenstinal tract (e.g. the cytochrome P450 3A enzyme), which subsequently increases the bioavailability, depending on the amount consumed, and an individual's susceptibility (Bailey *et al.* 1998). It has not been established whether the interaction between grapefruit juice and wafarin is significant. A study in which patients on warfarin were given grapefruit juice three times daily for a week had no effect on their prothrombin time measurements (Sullivan *et al.* 1998).

Similarly, with cranberry juice there have been ancedontal reports of the beverage increasing the antithrombotic effects of warfarin (Suvarna *et al.* 2003; Grant 2004; Rindone *et al.* 2006). It has been speculated that a natural component of cranberry juice inhibits the activity of the enzyme (cytochrome P450-2C9) responsible for the metabolism of warfarin, but this has not been credibly established (Greenblatt *et al.* 2005). Based on a total of 12 inconsistent case reports of suspected cranberry–warfarin interaction, the United Kingdom Committee on the Safety of Medicines (CSM) advised:

> Patients taking warfarin should avoid taking cranberry juice or other cranberry products unless the health benefits are considered to outweigh the risks.
>
> *(CSM 2004)*

Supporters in the cranberry camp have disputed this statement, citing a lack of evidence and highlighting the numerous underlying patient factors for loss of INR control in the published case reports, such as serious illness, dietary change and use of other medications (Greenblatt 2006). Studies of possible interactions are ongoing, and the latest evidence suggests that cranberry juice has no effect on the enzymes responsible for the metabolism of warfarin or on INR (Greenblatt *et al.* 2006; Zhaoping *et al.* 2006; Lilija *et al.* 2007).

Conflicting opinions make it difficult to advise patients, and until further data is available it is suggested that patients of VKA avoid consuming excessive amounts of either cranberry or grapefruit juice, but a modest intake is acceptable.

Bleeding complications of VKA therapy

The major concern with the use of anticoagulant therapy is the risk of bleeding. VKAs cause more fatal side-effects (virtually all related to bleeding complications) than any other drug in absolute numbers (Anonymous 1991). Major bleeding, which includes that leading to death, hospitalization or intracranial haemorrhage, has been reported in 1.2–8.1% of patients during each year of long-term warfarin therapy (Levine *et al.* 2001).

The major determinants of bleeding are the intensity and length of therapy. Studies show that bleeding risk increases as the INR increases (Palareti *et al.* 1996). The intensity of anticoagulation is the most important risk factor for intracranial haemorrhage, with the risk dramatically increasing with an INR >4.0, especially in patients aged over 75 years (Hylek *et al.* 1994).

Patient characteristics can also affect bleeding risk, as can the use of other drugs that interfere with haemostasis. Multiple studies have shown that elderly patients have an increased frequency of bleeding on warfarin therapy (Levine *et al.* 2001). Previous gastrointestinal bleeding is another risk factor, as are specific comorbid diseases, including hypertension, cerebrovascular disease, serious heart disease, renal insufficiency and malignancy (Levine *et al.* 2001).

Bleeding risk is greatest in the first three months after starting treatment, and risk factors can be additive (Baker *et al.* 2004). Many bleeding episodes are not clinically significant and patients should be reassured that minor nosebleeds, bruising and excessive bleeding after shaving is commonplace and not serious (Fitzmaurice *et al.* 2002). Bleeding from the renal or gastrointestinal tract often indicates an underlying lesion and warrants thorough investigation (Landefeld *et al.* 1993).

Warfarin reversal

If patients taking VKAs become over-anticoagulated or experience significant bleeding while on therapy, the effects may need to be reversed. The risk of bleeding increases noticeably once the INR is greater than 4. Management decisions, as always, need to be made on a case-by-case basis; however, guidelines for the management of non-therapeutic INRs are outlined in Table 7.4.

The first step is to discontinue further doses of warfarin therapy. If the effect is excessive, agents to counteract the anticoagulant effect may be needed, such as vitamin K followed by infusion of coagulation factors in the form of a prothrombin complex concentrate (PCC) and fresh frozen plasma (FFP).

Table 7.4 Guidelines for the management of non-therapeutic INRs

Clinical setting	Action
INR above therapeutic range but <5.0	Lower or omit the next dose of warfarin
No significant bleeding	Monitor frequently and resume therapy at an appropriately adjusted dose when INR therapeutic. If INR only minimally raised then dose reduction may not be necessary
INR 5.0–9.0	Stop warfarin therapy
No significant bleeding	If high risk of bleeding (GI disease, concomitant antiplatelet therapy, low platelet count, a major surgical procedure in preceding 2 weeks), give vitamin K (1.0–2.5 mg orally or 0.5–1.0 mg intravenously). If rapid reversal is required, e.g. for surgery, give 2–4 mg oral vitamin K and expect INR to reduce within 24 hours. Monitor INR frequently. Vitamin K effect on INR should be expected within 6–12 hours. Resume warfarin at reduced dose once INR therapeutic
INR >9.0	Stop warfarin therapy
Bleeding absent	Give vitamin K (2.5–5.0 mg orally or 1.0 mg intravenously) and measure INR in 6–12 hours. If high risk of bleeding, give 1.0 mg vitamin K intravenously. Consider PCC and fresh frozen plasma. Measure INR in 6–12 hours. Resume warfarin at a reduced dose once INR <5.0
Any clinically significant bleeding	Stop warfarin therapy
With an elevated INR	Give 5–10 mg vitamin K intravenously, supplemented with fresh frozen plasma (150–300 ml), prothrombin complex concentrate or recombinant factor VIIa. For persistent INR elevation, repeat vitamin K administration every 12 hours

(Adapted from Kearon *et al.* 2008; Ansell *et al.* 2001)

Vitamin K

Vitamin K1 (also called phylloquinone or phytomenadione) was discovered in 1929, when Danish scientist Henrik Dam noted haemorrhages in chickens fed a cholesterol-depleted diet. The bleeding defects were not corrected when cholesterol was reintroduced to the diet. The substance eventually found responsible for this was named the 'coagulation vitamin' (or 'Koagulationsvitamin') by German scientist Edward

Adelbert Doisy, hence the name Vitamin K (MacCorquodale *et al.* 1939).

Vitamin K can be administered both orally and intravenously. Intramuscular and subcutaneous administration are not recommended, since the response is unpredictable and occasionally delayed. Intramuscular injection poses the risk of haematoma formation and has been shown to have 'depot' characteristics, which can interfere with later recommencement of warfarin therapy (Whitling *et al.* 1998; Baker *et al.* 2004).

Oral vitamin K is the treatment of choice unless rapid anticoagulation is needed, and should be administered at a dose that will lower the INR to a safe but not subtherapeutic level (see Table 7.4). The intravenous route may be associated with anaphylactic reactions, so a slow administration is advised (O'Reilly *et al.* 1995). INR is usually normalized within 24 hours of administration of an i.v. dose of 5–10 mg vitamin K (Hirsh *et al.* 2003). Larger doses of vitamin K have been associated with some resistance to re-anticoagulation with warfarin; this can be avoided by giving smaller doses (Baker *et al.* 2004).

In a recent study of over-anticoagulated patients, low-dose vitamin K did lower the INR but did not appear to reduce bleeding, which supports the practice of treating patients with an INR in the 4.5–10.0 range with warfarin withdrawal alone (Crowther *et al.* 2009).

Prothrombin complex concentrate (PCC) and fresh frozen plasma (FFP)

PCCs are freeze-dried powder preparations of coagulation factors II, IX and X and low levels of factor VII, which are prepared from human plasma. Fresh frozen plasma is also obtained from the blood of voluntary donors but is separated and frozen within 8 hours of collection (therefore posing a greater infection risk than PCC) and contains all coagulation factors in variable quantities (Makris *et al.* 1997).

For patients with clinically significant bleeding who require a more immediate reversal of the anticoagulant effect of warfarin, PCC and FFP may be required. Vitamin K1 takes up to 24 hours to exert its full effects on the INR. PCCs can reverse warfarin anticoagulation immediately by providing adequate concentrations of the vitamin K-dependent clotting factors. However, the effects are only temporary and the British Committee for Standards in Haematology (BCSH) recommend that PCCs should be given in conjunction with 5–10 mg i.v. vitamin K to sustain the reversal in patients with life-threatening bleeding (BCSH 2004). PCCs have also been reported to show a thrombogenic effect.

PCCs should be used as first choice, but are not always readily available in all United Kingdom hospitals (Evans *et al.* 2008), therefore FFP must be used. FFP for warfarin reversal is not ideal, since it poses the risk of transfusion infections, requires large volumes of fluid and has a delay in action. Due to the variable content of vitamin K-dependent clotting factors in FFP, the efficacy is reduced. However, it can be used when immediate correction of INR is required and PCCs are not available (Makris *et al.* 1997). A comparison of PCC and FFP can be found in Table 7.5.

Table 7.5 Comparison of PCC and FFP

	Prothrombin complex concentrate (PCC)	**Fresh frozen plasma (FFP)**
What is it?	Prepared from plasma, a sterile, freeze-dried powder containig the vitamin K-dependent coagulation factors. Can be administered rapidly without the need for thawing	A source of all the coagulation factors. Separated from donor blood within hours of collection and frozen (thawing required prior to use)
Contraindications	In patients showing signs of thrombosis or disseminated intravascular coagulation	Not to be used when more effective alternatives available, such as vitamin K or specific factor concentrates
Availability	Not as widely available as FFP, but stocked in many hospitals or available from relevant blood service. No need to consider ABO group	Available in all ABO groups and should be ABO group compatible with patient's red cells (or use AB plasma)
Considerations for use	Allergies reported with PCC use. Predisposition to thrombosis, DIC and myocardial infarction	Allergic reactions and volume overload are common adverse events. Potential for transmission of blood-borne infection, transfusion-related acute lung injury and other transfusion reactions

(Data adapted from: Baker *et al.* 2004; Dickneite *et al.* 2009)

Case study 7.1: the accidental overdose

A 79 year-old female was brought into the emergency department by her granddaughter who suspects she has taken an overdose of her warfarin. She has only recently been diagnosed with a PE and commenced warfarin therapy a week earlier, the usual dose being 4 mg and 5 mg on alternating days. She contacted her grand-daughter this afternoon after realizing that she had erroneously taken four 5 mg tablets instead of four 1 mg tablets. The patient is haemodynamically stable, denies any bleeding or bruising and states that she is feeling well in herself. She is alert and orientated and says she mixed up the pill containers because she couldn't find her reading glasses. She is asking whether she can go home and wait until her next appointment at the anticoagulation clinic in a weeks time to have her INR taken.

How will you advise the patient?

Although the patient does not fit the criteria for a major bleed (see Box 7.5), she cannot wait a week before having her INR checked; 20 mg warfarin is a significant dose and, remember, the effects of the medication are delayed, so even if her INR is within range initially, if she leaves without further monitoring and advice in place she could develop problems at home. You should explain this to her, then take

Box 7.5 Management of major/life-threatening bleed (intracranial, intraocular, compartment syndrome, pericardial, active bleeding and shock)

- Urgent clinical assessment.
- Check FBC, INR, APTT, fibrinogen (and D-dimer if possibility of DIC).
- Contact a haematologist.
- Stop warfarin.
- Reverse anticoagulation with 5 mg slow intravenous vitamin K and PCC, 30 units/kg (discuss with haematologist – if evidence of DIC, PCC may be contraindicated; can exacerbate underlying hypercoagulable state)
- If PCC unavailable, FFP 15 ml/kg can be used with 5 mg slow intravenous vitamin K.

bloods for FBC and coagulation studies. The patient's FBC comes back unremarkable and the INR is 2.6 (target INR is 2.5, on warfarin for prior VTE).

Do you think vitamin K is indicated in this patient?

A management plan for non-therapeutic INRs is outlined in Table 7.4. In this patient with an INR of <5 with no signs of bleeding, established treatment protocols would recommend that the next dose of warfarin be omitted and the INR monitored until it is in the therapeutic range. However, this case is somewhat unusual in its presentation. Most patients do not present within hours of taking a warfarin overdose, therefore warfarin reversal strategies (which are based on the fact that onset of coagulation can be delayed for 48–72 hours) are of limited use in this scenario. Anecdotal evidence suggests that administration of oral vitamin K in such a case will prevent the anticipated rise in INR, thus reducing the risk of bleeding complications, although this is not widely established (Cryder *et al.* 2008). Each case should be assessed individually to weigh up the risk of bleeding against the risk of thrombosis, and discussion with a senior colleague is advised if there is any doubt. It would be reasonable to withhold vitamin K, admit this lady for a period of observation and monitoring of her INR and have warfarin reversal agents to hand should she develop signs of bleeding.

Anticoagulation and surgery

Managing patients who require surgery who are also on long-term warfarin therapy is a difficult area, which involves balancing the risk of bleeding from the surgery with the increased risk of VTE associated with prolonged immobility during the procedure. During the first few months after a thromboembolic event, the high risk of recurrence makes even a temporary reduction in warfarin therapy undesirable (Schulman 2003). If anticoagulants must be stopped for surgery soon after VTE, a vena cava filter can be placed to minimize the risk of life-threatening PE (Gallus *et al.* 2000).

Minor operations such as simple dental procedures, soft tissue aspirations and dermatological procedures, which all carry a low risk of bleeding, do not require interruption to warfarin therapy if the INR is within the therapeutic range (Douketis *et al.* 2008). For oral surgery, continuation of warfarin is safer if combined with a mouth rinse of 5% tranexamic acid solution four times daily for a week (Ramstrom *et al.* 1993).

For most major surgical procedures and high-risk endoscopy, the intensity of anticoagulation should be reduced to prevent bleeding and restarted as soon as circumstances allow, protecting against the increased risk of thromboembolism associated with surgery (Schulman 2003). After warfarin is stopped, it takes approximately four days for the INR to reach 1.5, which is the level at which surgery can be safely performed. It then takes another three days for the INR to reach 2.0 once it is restarted postoperatively (Kearon *et al.* 1997). Patients need to have a normal state of coagulation during surgery, so some period without anticoagulation (and thus an increased risk of thromboembolism) is unavoidable. Strategies for adjusting therapy are outlined in Table 7.6. For most patients warfarin can be withheld for five days prior

Table 7.6 Anticoagulation therapy during major surgical procedures

	Patients at low risk of VTE	Patients at high risk of VTE
Prior to surgery	Withhold warfarin 4–5 days prior to surgery If INR >2 the night before surgery, give 1–5mg intravenous vitamin K	Withhold warfarin 4–5 days prior to surgery 2–3 days before surgery give daily or twice daily doses of either IV unfractionated heparin (UH)or SC low molecular weight heparin (LMWH)
	If INR >1.5 on day of surgery, defer it. If urgent, give PCC (or FFP if PCC not available)	If using LMWH, the last dose should be at least 24 hours before surgery. If using UH, it should be stopped 4–6 hours before surgery
After surgery	Start warfarin on the day of surgery at the previous maintenance dose Start thromboprophylaxis as per usual practice	Restart warfarin as soon as possible after the procedure Start UH (aiming to prolong the APTT by 1.5 times) or LMWH (at a thromboprophylactic dose) 12–24 hours postoperatively Fully anticoagulate the patient with warfarin 72 hours postoperatively if there is no evidence of bleeding Stop UH or LMWH therapy 48 hours after target INR is reached

(Adapted from Kearon *et al.* 1997; Douketis *et al.* 2008; Baker *et al.* 2004)

to elective surgery and the risk of thrombosis should be assessed (Baker *et al.* 2004). Patients at high risk of VTE should receive 'bridging anticoagulation' with heparin during the temporary cessation of their warfarin (Douketis *et al.* 2008). The INR should be measured the day before surgery to ensure adequate reversal. If the INR is 1.8 or higher, there is the option of administering a small dose of vitamin K. Warfarin should be restarted as soon as possible following the procedure (Kearon *et al.* 1997).

Case study 7.2: warfarin and surgery

A 54 year-old lady who is on long-term warfarin therapy for recurrent DVT is due to undergo elective surgery for repair of an incisional hernia.

What advice would you give her prior to the procedure regarding her warfarin therapy?

A VTE risk assessment should be carried out. We know she is on warfarin for recurrent VTE but it is important to determine when the last episode of VTE occurred and whether or not it occurred in the presence of reversible risk factors. This patient should be advised to withhold warfarin therapy for five days prior to her procedure, until the INR falls to below 1.5. Since she is at high risk of VTE, she should commence heparin bridging therapy during the cessation of warfarin. Postprocedure warfarin should be restarted as soon as possible after the procedure. See Table 7.6 for more information.

How would her warfarin therapy be managed if she was undergoing a minor dental procedure?

Patients undergoing minor operations at low risk of bleeding generally do not need to discontinue warfarin therapy if their INR is within the therapeutic range. Her INR should be measured and for dental procedures, continuation of warfarin is safer if combined with a mouth rinse of a 5% solution of tranexamic acid four times daily for a week.

The same patient develops a small bowel obstruction and must be taken to theatre urgently. How would her warfarin therapy be managed in this instance?

Complete and rapid reversal of anticoagulation prior to emergency surgery can be achieved with a factor concentrate or with fresh frozen plasma. Vitamin K can be used in semi-urgent situations, for example if surgery must be done within 24–96 hours. High doses can cause postoperative resistance to warfarin, so smaller doses should be used if anticoagulation is expected to be started following the procedure. Vitamin K is not routinely used before elective surgery (Jaffer *et al.* 2003).

Warfarin and pregnancy

Warfarin can cross the placenta, so is contraindicated in pregnant patients due to the teratogenic effects of VKA. VKAs given between 6 and 12 weeks of gestation have induced the 'warfarin embryopathy syndrome', leading to midface and nasal hypoplasia, stippled epiphyses, hypoplasia of the digits, optic atrophy and mental impairment (Stevenson *et al.* 1980). It can also cause CNS haemorrhage in the fetus during any trimester. Warfarin is not contraindicated during breast-feeding, since the concentration in breast milk is <25 ng/ml and is undetectable in the plasma of breast-fed infants (Orme *et al.* 1977). Heparins do not cross the placenta, so these problems are avoided (Sanson *et al.* 1999).

Other complications of VKA therapy

After bleeding episodes, skin necrosis is the next most common complication, occurring at a frequency of 1 in 5000 patients, typically females (Gallerani *et al.* 1995). Symptoms typically start within 3–10 days after initiating therapy and manifest as localized pain with a maculopapular rash, which progress within 48 hours to haemorrhagic lesions and necrosis, leaving an eschar which frequently requires plastic surgery. The reaction is thought to be due to a hypercoaguable state caused by depressed levels of protein C and protein S and an underlying deficiency of the two proteins, or use of a large loading dose of warfarin may accentuate this imbalance (Gallerani *et al.* 1995). Prompt delivery of vitamin K has been shown to avoid progression to skin necrosis.

'Purple toe syndrome' has been reported in a few patients commenced on warfarin, mainly in patients with underlying cardiac disorders, diabetes mellitus or peripheral vascular disease. It is thought to be due to cholesterol embolization from atherosclerotic plaques, which warfarin makes more friable and prone to embolize. Symptoms include burning pain in the toes with dark blue discoloration; sometimes the hands are involved too (Sallah *et al.* 1997).

Hypersensitivity reactions have been reported with warfarin use, mainly in the form of urticarial, itchy skin rashes. Less common reactions include eosinophilic pleurisy, vasculitis and, very rarely, toxic hepatitis (Schulman 2001).

Unfractionated heparin (UFH)

Heparin is a naturally occurring anticoagulant, discovered to have antithrombotic properties over 90 years ago (McLean 1916). It was named 'heparin' by William Howell due to the fact he isolated it from the liver. It has been used extensively as treatment for VTE for the past 50 years.

Pharmacokinetics

UFH is a glycosaminoglycan derived from pig intestine or bovine lung tissue. It is made up of chains of polysaccharides which vary in molecular weight in the range 3000–30 000 Daltons with a mean weight of 15 000 Daltons. The mass of a heparin molecule is an important determinant of its anticoagulant properties (Hirsh et al. 2004; Raskob et al. 2001). It has been established that the region of heparin responsible for anticoagulation is a unique pentasaccharide sequence that is only present in about one-third of UFH molecules (Choay et al. 1981).

Simply put, the anticoagulant effect of UFH occurs when it binds to antithrombin III, after which it is capable of inhibiting multiple steps in the coagulation cascade, involving mainly thrombin and factor Xa. Inactivation of thrombin prevents fibrin formation and also inhibits thrombin-induced activation of factors V and VIII (Hirsh et al. 2001a). The inhibition of thrombin by heparin is different from its inhibition of factor Xa. Thrombin inhibition requires heparin to first bind to antithrombin III. The smaller heparin molecules, which contain <18 saccharide units, are unable to bind to both thrombin and antithrombin III simultaneously. However, these smaller molecules can still augment the inhibition of factor Xa (see section on LMWH, below) (Raskob et al. 2001).

UFH can have unpredictable pharmacodynamics and pharmacokinetic properties because it also binds endothelial cells, platelet factor 4 and platelets (Hirsh et al. 2004). LMWHs do not have the same non-specific binding affinities and therefore have more predictable properties.

Heparin prolongs bleeding time in humans, increases vessel wall permeability, suppresses the proliferation of vascular smooth muscle cells and suppresses osteoblast formation while activating osteoclasts, which promotes bone loss (Hirsh et al. 2001a, 2004).

UFH is administered parenterally by either continuous intravenous (i.v.) infusion or subcutaneous (s.c.) injection. Given by the s.c. route, heparin has a lower bioavailability and less predictable pharmacological properties, and if an immediate anticoagulant effect is required the initial dose should be accompanied by an i.v. bolus injection, because the effect of s.c. heparin is delayed for 1–2 hours (Hirsh *et al.* 2001a; Kearon *et al.* 2008). Once it has entered the circulation, heparin binds to plasma proteins, macrophages and endothelial cells, which reduces its anticoagulant activity (Hirsh *et al.* 2004). Heparin is cleared renally and, due to its binding properties, its half-life varies depending on the dose administered, ranging from a half-life of 30 minutes following an i.v. bolus of 25 U/kg to 60 minutes with an i.v. bolus of 100 U/kg to 150 minutes with an i.v. bolus of 400 U/kg (Hirsh *et al.* 2004).

Indications

Heparin is the standard therapy for VTE and is widely used to treat patients with acute coronary syndromes to prevent mural thrombosis following myocardial infarction. It is used to prevent thrombosis during vascular surgery or angioplasty procedures and to prevent thrombi during cardiopulmonary bypass surgery. Heparin is also used in the prevention of VTE in medical patients and following surgery (Raskob *et al.* 2001). Heparin and LMWH do not cross the placenta and so can be used as alternatives to warfarin during pregnancy.

Initiation and duration

The anticoagulant response to heparin in patients with thromboembolic disorders is known to vary, so it is standard practice to adjust the dose and monitor its effect, usually by measurement of the activated partial thromboplastin time (APTT; see below). The risk of heparin-induced bleeding increases with the dose administered and with concomitant thrombolytic and glycoprotein IIb/IIIa therapy (Hirsh *et al.* 2001). A relationship has been noted between the dose of heparin given and both its efficacy and its safety, so the dose must be adjusted, usually based on the patient's weight by way of treatment nomograms (Hirsh *et al.* 2004).

Current ACCP recommendations in patients with VTE are that if i.v. heparin is the drug of choice, an initial bolus of 80 U/kg (or 5000 U) should be given followed by a continuous infusion, starting at 18 U/kg/hour (or 1300 U/hour), which is monitored and adjusted to maintain an appropriate APTT prolongation, as outlined by the nomograms below.

If s.c. heparin is given for acute VTE, the ACCP advises an initial dose of 250 U/kg (or 17 500 U) twice daily, with dose adjustment according to APTT. If APTT is not being monitored, then the s.c. dose given should be 333 U/kg initially, followed by a twice daily dose of 250 U/kg, rather than non-weight-based dosing (Kearon *et al.* 2008).

In patients with VTE, heparin (either UFH or LMWH) treatment should continue for at least five days, while VKA therapy is being initiated until the INR is >2.0 for at least 24 hours (Kearon *et al.* 2008).

Monitoring

UFH requires frequent monitoring, due to its unpredictable anticoagulant effect. The APTT (also known as the partial thromboplastin time, PTT) is the most convenient and frequently used method of monitoring this. It measures the efficacy of both the intrinsic and common pathways of the coagulation cascade. APTT should be measured 6 hours after the bolus dose of heparin and the continuous dose of heparin adjusted according to the result (Hirsh *et al.* 2001a). There are many dose-adjustment nomograms in use, such as the one outlined in Table 7.7. It is best to use the protocol in place at your own institution, since the APTT measurements can vary between laboratories, depending on the reagents used (Brill-Edwards *et al.* 1993).

In general, clotting should occur in 25–35 seconds. In a patient taking heparin, clotting takes up to two and a half times longer. APTT results are given as a ratio of the result compared to the usual normal values of a patient not taking anticoagulants, i.e. a therapeutic range for heparin is usually expressed as an APTT of 1.5–2.5 to 'normal' value,

Table 7.7 Weight-based nomogram for heparin dosing

Initial dose	80 U/kg bolus, then 18 U/kg/hour infusion
aPTT <35 seconds (<1.2 × control)	80 U/kg bolus, then 4 U/kg/hour infusion
aPTT 35–45 seconds (1.2–1.5 × control)	40 U/kg bolus, then 2 U/kg/hour infusion
aPTT 46–70 seconds (1.5–2.3 × control)	No change
aPTT 71–90 seconds (2.3–3 × control)	Decrease infusion rate by 2 U/kg/hour
aPTT >90 seconds (>3 × control)	Interrupt infusion for 1 hour, then decrease infusion rate by 3 U/kg/hour

(Adapted from Raschke *et al.* 1996)

but again this range varies from institution to institution. To allow for differences between laboratories, the therapeutic APTT range can be calibrated for each specific reagent used by determining the APTT values that correspond with therapeutic heparin levels (equivalent to 0.3–0.7 IU/ml when assayed for factor Xa inhibition) (Hirsh *et al.* 2004). In patients receiving high doses of heparin, such as those undergoing cardiac bypass surgery, the activated clotting time (ACT) is often used to monitor the effects, since the APPT is often prolonged beyond the measurable upper limit (Raskob *et al.* 2001).

Heparin monitoring is likely to become less problematic in the future as LMWH replaces UFH for most indications (Hirsh 1998).

Complications and contraindications

Side effects of heparin therapy include:

- Bleeding.
- Thrombocytopenia.
- Osteoporosi.
- Raised transaminase levels [deranged liver function tests (LFTs)].
- Hypersensitivity and skin reactions.
- Hyperkalemia due to hypoaldosteronism (rare).
- Alopecia (rare).

Bleeding

Similar to warfarin therapy, those at risk of bleeding include the elderly, those with a history of gastrointestinal or genitourinary bleeding, patients who have undergone recent surgery and those with a predisposition to bleeding. The rates of major bleeding reporting from i.v. heparin treatment are in the range 0–7% (Raskob *et al.* 2001).

Treatment is according to clinical severity and APPT level (Hirsh *et al.* 2001a). If bleeding develops while on UFH, the heparin should be stopped. While the half-life of UFH is dose-dependent, the effects can last up to three hours, so observation of the clinical condition and serial APPT measurements should be taken to determine when the infusion can be restarted.

In severe bleeding, the anticoagulant effects of heparin can be rapidly neutralized by an i.v. bolus of protamine. Protamine is a basic protein derived from fish sperm that binds to heparin to form a stable salt; 1 mg protamine sulphate will neutralize approximately 100 units of UFH. If an i.v. bolus of 5000 units of heparin were given, a dose of 50 mg protamine would be required (given slowly i.v.). Doses >50 mg are rarely required because heparin is cleared quickly from plasma, with a half-life of approximately 60 minutes. After s.c. doses of heparin repeated small doses of protamine may be required, due to prolonged heparin absorption from the s.c. depot and because of the short half-life of protamine (Raskob *et al.* 2001). The APPT can be used to monitor the effectiveness of the antiheparin therapy (Hirsh *et al.* 2001a). Allergic reactions have been documented with protamine and patients with a known allergy to fish, who may be more susceptible to reaction, can be given corticosteroids and antihistamines prior to treatment (Hirsh *et al.* 2001a).

Other methods to neutralize the effects of UFH include the use of hexadimethrine, heparinase, platelet factor 4, extracorporeal heparin removal devices and synthetic protamine, however these therapies are not widely available (Hirsh J *et al.* 2001a).

Thrombocytopenia

Two types of heparin-induced thrombocytopenia (HIT) have been described. Type I is early non-immune throbocytopenia, which usually occurs within 1–5 days of initiating therapy. It is due to platelet aggregation and is usually transient and benign (Raskob *et al.* 2001). Type II is caused by IgG or IgM antibody formation directed against UFH and platelet factor 4. This causes platelet activation to occur, which causes thrombocytopenia and a tendency for thrombosis (Greinacher *et al.* 1994). Clinically, type II HIT can cause extension of VTE, skin necrosis (Figure 7.1) and arterial thrombosis, complications which have been

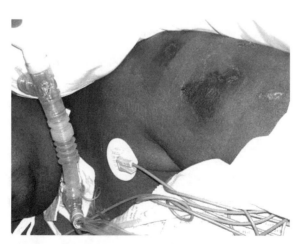

Figure 7.1 Heparin-induced skin necrosis. Included with the permission of The King's Thrombosis Centre.

associated with limb amputation and a high mortality rate (Warkentin *et al.* 1996). In these instances, heparin should be discontinued. Protamine is not effective against the immune-mediated response. The platelet count usually returns to normal in 4–6 days. In those patients who still require anticoagulation, the options are danaparoid sodium (which exhibits anti factor Xa activity) or recombinant hirudin (see below).

Osteoporosis

Osteoporosis may occur as a side-effect of long-term heparin therapy of more than three months, usually manifesting as non-specific low back pain. Patients may report spontaneous fractures of the ribs and vertebrae The incidence of symptomatic fractures is estimated to be 2% and it is thought that up to one-third of patients on long-term heparin therapy may have subclinical reductions in bone density (Raskob *et al.* 2001). Osteopenia is caused by the binding of heparin to osteoblasts (Hirsh *et al.* 2001a).

Low molecular weight heparin (LMWH)

LMWH is largely taking over from heparin as the agent of choice for both prevention and treatment of VTE, for the reasons outlined in Table 7.8. LMWHs are as effective and safe as UFH and more convenient, although they are more expensive. However, in the long-term, use of

Table 7.8 Advantages of LMWH over UFH

Pharmacological effects	Clinical benefits
Fast, predictable SC absorption	More reliable level of anticoagulation
More stable dose–response	Removes need for monitoring
Resistance to platelet factor 4 inhibition	Decreased incidence of thrombocytopenia
Decreased antiheparin antibody production	Greater antithrombotic effect
Less antithrombin activity	Potential to reduce bleeding
Ease of administration	Absence of 'rebound' and makes outpatient therapy possible
	Reduced binding to osteoclasts, leading to less bone loss

(Adapted from Hirsh 1998; Hirsh *et al.* 2001a; Hyers 2003)

LMWH allows for outpatient management and reduced hospital stay, which ultimately make it the more economical option (Hirsh *et al.* 2001a).

Pharmacokinetics

LMWH is derived from UFH through depolymerization using an enzymatic process, which results in smaller molecules, 4000–6000 Daltons in size (Raskob *et al.* 2001). LMWH exerts its anticoagulant effects in a similar way to UFH (see above) by activating antithrombin III. The shorter chain lengths mean that LMWHs cannot bind simultaneously to antithrombin III and thrombin, resulting in a reduced ability to inactivate thrombin and an enhanced ability for inactivating factor Xa.

A clinically useful feature of LMWH is that is does not bind as readily as UFH to plasma proteins, endothelial cells and macrophages, which results in more predictable pharmacological properties and a longer half-life. LMWH also has a high bioavailability, which allows for s.c. administration of fixed doses without the need for laboratory monitoring (Raskob *et al.* 2001).

The anticoagulant response to a fixed dose of LMWH is related to body weight, therefore treatment regimens are based on units per kg body weight. LMWH is cleared by the kidneys, so it follows that clearance is reduced in patients with renal failure and toxicity can occur. Monitoring of anti-Xa activity can be carried out in renal patients as a marker for determining the degree of decreased ability for thrombosis, to guide dosing and to monitor potential accumulation of the drug and potential risks for bleeding (Laposta *et al.* 1998). This is not routinely done in practice because the marginal improvement in clinical outcome is offset by the added inconvenience and expense (Hirsh *et al.* 2001a). Peak anti Xa levels occur 4 hours after a therapeutic dose of s.c. LMWH and peak levels above the upper limit of the therapeutic range (0.6–1.0 IU/ml) may be associated with an increased risk for bleeding (Hirsh *et al.* 2004).

Indications

The major uses of LMWH are:

- Treatment of VTE.
- Prevention of postoperative VTE.
- Prevention of VTE in patients with acute medical diseases.
- Acute coronary syndrome.
- Prevention of coagulation during extracorporal circulation during renal dialysis.

Table 7.9 Commercially available LMWH and methods of preparation

Generic name	Trade name	Method of preparation
Ardeparin	Normiflo	Perioxidative depolymerization
Dalteparin	Fragmin	Nitrous acid depolymerization
Enoxaparin sodium	Clexane/Lovenox	Benzylation followed by alkaline depolymerization
Nadroparin calcium	Fraxiparin	Nitrous acid depolymerization
Reviparin	Clivarine	Nitrous acid depolymerization
Tinzaparin	Innohep	Enzymatic depolymerization with heparinase

(Adapted from Hirsh *et al.* 2001a)

Dosing

The various LMWHs approved for use in Europe, Canada and the United States are listed in Table 7.9. Due to the differences in preparation, they differ slightly in their pharmacological properties and anticoagulant profile.

Weight-adjusting dosing is the recommended practice and due to the predictable response of LMWH, APPT monitoring is not required. Data regarding LMWH dosing in obese patients is limited, but trials carried out in patients with acute coronary syndrome suggest that LMWH dosing can be based on total body weight, up to a maximum of 160 kg. Patients heavier than this should be considered for monitoring of anti-Xa activity (Cohen *et al.* 2001). A recent study by Bazinet *et al.* (2005) suggests that, based on anti-Xa, no dosage adjustments are required in obese patients; however, further research is required.

In patients with chronic renal failure, serious adverse bleeding incidents have been reported with the use of LMWHs administered at fixed weight doses without monitoring (Farooq *et al.* 2004). There appears to be an increased risk for haemorrhagic complications in patients with renal failure, irrespective of the form of anticoagulation therapy used. Studies have shown that bleeding complications with UFH and LMWH are comparable (Thorevska *et al.* 2004); however, unlike UFH, the anticoagulant effects of LMWH cannot be completely reversed.

Due to concerns regarding accumulation of LMWH and bleeding in patients with renal impairment, the College of American Pathologists recommend UFH instead of LMWH in patients with a creatinine clearance of 30 ml/min or less or, alternatively, monitoring of anti-Xa activity if LMWH is used (Laposta *et al.* 1998). More recent data suggest that adjusted doses of LMWH in renal impairment may reduce the risk for bleeding events, but further research is needed (Lim *et al.* 2006). Recent guidelines regarding weight-adjusted dosing are outlined in Box 7.6.

Box 7.6 LMWH weight-based dosing for treatment of VTE (enoxaparin/fondaparinux)

For treatment of VTE (must overlap with warfarin for at least 5 days and until INR is within therapeutic range for 2 consecutive days)

Enoxaparin

- Once daily dosing, 1.5 mg per kg every day.
- Twice daily dosing, 1 mg per kg every 12 hours.

Fondiparinux

Weight <50 kg, 5 mg once daily.
Weight 50–100 kg, 7.5 mg once daily.
Weight >100 kg, 10 mg once daily.

Modified management in patients with risk factors

Risk factor	Recommended management	Anticoagulant
BMI >35	Monitor anti-Xa levels*	Enoxaparin
Weight <50 kg		Fondaparinux
Pregnancy	Monitor anti-Xa levels*	Enoxaparin
	Consult haematologist	
Renal insufficiency (CrCl <30 ml/min)	Preference is to use UFH. If LMWH used, reduce dose by 50%	Enoxaparin Fondaparinux

*Check anti-factor Xa 4 hours after dose given. Once patient has a therapeutic level, measure anti-factor Xa once per week 4 hours post dose. Target peak anti-Xa level with twice daily enoxaparin is 0.6–1.2 U/ml and with once daily enoxaparin and fondaparinux is 1.0–2.0 U/ml.

Patients should have platelet count and serum creatinine monitoring. Suspect HIT if platelet count falls by >50% *or* a thrombotic event occurs between days 5 and 14 following initiation of heparin.

(Adapted from Hirsh *et al.* 2008)

Complications and contraindications

The key advantages of LMWH over UFH have already been outlined, namely the convenience of once or twice daily dosing with s.c. injections and a reduction in toxic effects, such as HIT and osteoporosis. However, LMWH still has reported complications.

The risk of HIT is lower than with UFH but remains a concern, and reported side-effects include local skin reactions and skin necrosis. Bleeding remains a side-effect of LMWH and protamine will neutralize the antithrombin activity of LMWH but has little effect on the anti-factor Xa activity (Hirsh *et al.* 2004).

In clinical situations where the antithrombotic effect of LMWH needs to be neutralized, it is advised that protamine is given; 1 mg protamine can neutralize 1 mg enoxaparin and 100 units dalteparin (or 100 anti-factor Xa units LMWH). A second dose may be considered in patients who continue bleeding and the use of FFP and packed red blood cells should also be considered, with haematological consultation (Hirsh J *et al.* 2004).

Case study 7.3: an aversion to hospitals

A 60 year-old gentleman attends the emergency department with a swollen right calf. He tells you that he was discharged from hospital 3 months ago following a right knee replacement operation and hasn't been as mobile as usual since then. He is otherwise in good health, with no past medical history. DVT is diagnosed and you explain the treatment to him. His main concern at present is his wife at home, who he doesn't want to stay in the house by herself without him. He is insistent that he is not going to stay in hospital for any further monitoring.

This patient may be a candidate for outpatient LMWH therapy, depending on the policy in place at your particular hospital. First, you need to determine his suitability. Exclusion criteria for outpatient LMWH therapy (Yeager *et al.* 1999) include:

- Clinical evidence or suspicion of progression to PE (many units now also have outpatient PE protocols, so some patients may still be suitable for home management, depending on the clinical picture. This serves as a reminder to be aware of clinical deterioration).
- Conditions that increase the risk of bleeding.
- High risk of recurrent thrombosis.

- Likelihood of non-compliance.
- Unavailability for follow-up.
- Inadequate home support system.

He should be given detailed verbal and written information regarding his treatment and have access to hospital staff who can help him, should he need further advice. Warfarin treatment should overlap with LMWH therapy for 5–7 days and then warfarin will be continued alone for a duration dependent on the reasons for anticoagulation. It is important that he understands the dosing, how to manage missed doses, overdoses and any drug interactions. Advise him on the importance of follow-up and returning for monitoring of his INR. The patient should be made aware of the signs and symptoms of recurrent thrombosis and bleeding events and should be advised where to seek help and what to do should this happen. A full explanation on injection technique is given in Chapter 8 (see Figure 8.6, p. 210).

Protocols may differ between hospitals, but baseline bloods should be taken prior to starting anticoagulation to include haemoglobin and platelet count, APPT and PT/INR. An INR should be taken on the third day of therapy and again daily until the LMWH therapy is discontinued (Yeager *et al.* 1999). LMWH is usually discontinued after at least 5 days of therapy have been administered and once the INR is at the desired target for 24 hours (Kearon *et al.* 2008). A platelet count should be repeated on the fifth day of therapy. Once again, refer to the protocol in place at your own unit, as there may be variations. Advise him to look out for side-effects and episodes of recurrent thrombosis and ensure that follow-up is arranged.

Newer anticoagulants

Factor Xa inhibitors

Fondaparinux is a small synthetic pentasaccharide consisting entirely of the antithrombin-binding sequence of heparin. Its principal anticoagulant effect is as a catalyst to enhance the antithrombin-dependent inhibition of factor Xa, which subsequently inhibits thrombin generation (Hyers 2003).

Fondaparinux does not affect platelet function and exhibits no non-specific binding to plasma proteins. It is rapidly absorbed following s.c. administration, with a long half-life of approximately 17 hours, which allows for once-daily dosing with a rapid onset of action and no need for monitoring (Hyers 2003). Dose adjustments are necessary in patients with renal insufficiency and it should be avoided in those with renal failure (Weitz *et al.* 2004).

Fondaparinux is currently approved for the prevention of VTE after major orthopaedic surgery, showing a reduction in VTE compared to LMWH, with no difference in clinically relevant bleeding episodes (Turpie *et al.* 2001). It has also been shown to be equally as effective as LMWH and UFH in the initial treatment of patients with VTE; however, there is currently a lack of sufficient information on the safety of its use. Further research is awaited (Nijkeuter *et al.* 2004).

Danaparoid

Danaparoid is a heparinoid LMWH which inhibits factor Xa. Its main use in practice is in patients with HIT (Magnani 1993); it appears to be safe in pregnancy and does not cross the placenta (Greinacher *et al.* 1993). The major disadvantage of danaparoid is its prolonged half-life and the lack of a reversing agent. It is not available in the United States but can be obtained in Canada and Europe.

Direct thrombin inhibitors (DTI)

Hirudin is a 65 amino acid polypeptide produced by the salivary gland of the medical leech, and was the first DTI to be used medically. Recombinant hirudin was subsequently developed using DNA technology- and several other DTIs followed on from this, including drugs such as bivalirudin, dabigatran and ximelagatran (Raskob *et al.* 2001). Rivaroxaban is an oral direct inhibitor of factor Xa and thrombin, which acts for 24 hours, offering once-daily dosing and the potential for no monitoring (Graff *et al.* 2007).

Unlike heparin, DTIs are capable of inhibiting both circulating thrombin and clot-bound thrombin. They do not bind to plasma proteins, neither do they require antithrombin III as a cofactor and they do not inhibit other coagulation pathway enzymes; they therefore have a more predictable anticoagulant effect. DTIs are currently indicated in patients with HIT, since they do not cause thrombocytopenia (Warkentin *et al.* 2004).

Despite the convenience of DTIs, in that monitoring is not needed and thrombocytopenia is avoided, their major drawback is an increased risk of bleeding (Hyers 2003).

Other anticoagulants

Many new anticoagulants are under development, such as nematode anticoagulant peptide c2, which has the ability to be administered every two days (Weitz *et al.* 2004). The ideal treatment will have properties such as once-daily dosing and oral administration, without the need for monitoring or dose adjustment. Ideally, these agents will have improved pharmacodynamic profiles and targeted activity at single points in the coagulation cascade to reduce the side-effect profile. For a more detailed profile of the newer agents under development, please refer to the ACCP article by Weitz *et al.* (2004).

Conclusion

The management of VTE through the use of anticoagulants has proved to be an effective means of reducing further thrombotic episodes. However, initiating patients on anticoagulants requires consideration. Patients should be assessed for bleeding risk and their current state of health and concomitant use of medications needs to be considered. Patient education is key in ensuring that patients understand their treatment and the potential side-effects. Importance should be given to regular monitoring and awareness of how anything they consume can potentially affect their treatment. Newer anticoagulants are continually under development, and the ideal treatment will combine properties such as once-daily dosing and oral administration without the need for monitoring or dose adjustment.

References

Ageno W, Turpie AG (1998) A randomised comparison of a computer based dosing program with a manual system to monitor oral anticoagulant therapy. *Thrombosis Research* **91**: 237–240.

Albers GW, Dalen JE, Laupacis A *et al.* (2001) Antithrombotic therapy in atrial fibrillation. *Chest* **119**: 194–206S.

Anderson DR, Harrison L, Hirsh J (1993) Evaluation of a portable prothrombin time monitor for home use by patients who require long-term oral anticoagulant therapy. *Archives of Internal Medicine* **153**: 1441–1448.

Anonymous (1991) ADR reporting in Sweden in 1991. *Bulletin from the Swedish Adverse Drug Reaction Advisory Committee* **62**: 1.

Ansell J, Hirsh J, Dalen J *et al.* (2001) Managing oral anticoagulant therapy. *Chest* **119**: 22–38S.

Ascani A, Iorio A, Agnelli G (1999) Withdrawal of warfarin after deep vein thrombosis: effects of a low fixed dose on rebound thrombin generation. *Blood Coagulation and Fibrinolysis* **10**: 291–295.

Bailey DG, Malcolm J, Arnold O *et al.* (1998) Grapefruit juice–drug interactions. *British Journal of Clinical Pharmacology* **46**: 101–110.

Baker RI, Coughlin PB, Gallus AS *et al.* (2004) Warfarin reversal: consensus guidelines, on behalf of the Australasian Society of Thrombosis and Haemostasis. *Medical Journal of Australia* **181**: 492–497.

Bazinet A, Almanric K, Brunet C *et al.* (2005) Dosage of enoxaparin among obese and renal impairment patients. *Thrombosis Research* **116**: 41–50.

Blickstein D, Shaklai M, Inbal A (1991). Warfarin antagonism by avocado. *Lancet* **337**: 914–917.

Brandjes DPM, Heijboer H, Buller HR *et al.* (1992) Acenocoumarol and heparin compared with acenocoumarol alone in the initial treatment of proximal vein thrombosis. *New England Journal of Medicine* **327**: 1485–1489.

Brill-Edwards P, Ginsberg JS, Johnston M *et al.* (1993) Establishing a therapeutic range for heparin therapy. *Annals of Internal Medicine* **119**: 104–109.

British Committee for Standards in Haematology (BCSH) Blood Transfusion Task Force (2004) Guidelines for the use of fresh frozen plasma, cryoprecipitate and cryosupernatant. *British Journal of Haematology* **126**: 11–28.

British National Formulary (BNF) (2008) Royal Pharmaceutical Society of Great Britain. British Medical Journal Publishing Group, London.

Bussey HI, Tapson V, Cannon RO *et al.* (2005) NIH conference on dietary supplements, session V: opinions and research priorities. *Thrombosis Research* **117**: 155–169.

Cairns JA, Theroux P, Lewis HD Jr *et al.* (2001) Antithrombotic agents in coronary artery disease. *Chest* **119**(suppl): 228–252S [published correction appears in *Chest* **120**: 1427].

Campbell P, Robert G, Eaton V *et al.* (2001) Managing warfarin therapy in the community. *Australian Prescriber* **24**: 86–89.

Choay J, Lormeau JC, Petitou M *et al.* (1981) Structural studies on a biologically active hexasaccharide obtained from heparin. *Annals of the New York Academy of Science* **370**: 644–649.

Cohen M, Antman EM, Gurfinkel EP *et al.* (2001) The ESSENCE (Efficacy and Safety of Subcutaneous Enoxaparin in Non-Q wave Coronary Events) and TIMI 11B investigators: enoxaparin in unstable angina/non ST segment elevation myocardial infarction: treatment benefits in prespecified subgroups. *Journal of Thrombosis and Thrombolysis* **12**: 199–206.

Committee on Safety of Medicines, Medicines and Healthcare Products Regulatory Agency (2004) Interaction between warfarin and cranberry juice: new advice. *Current Problems in Pharmacovilgilance* **30**: 10.

Crowther MA, Ageno W, Garcia W *et al.* (2009) Oral vitamin K versus placebo to correct excessive anticoagulation in patients receiving warfarin. A randomized trial. *Annals of Internal Medicine* **150**: 293–300.

Cryder BT, Felczak MA, Rojszyk JD (2008) Management of an unintentional warfarin overdose with oral vitamin K in the outpatient setting prior to elevation of the International Normalized Ratio – case report. *Journal of Patient Safety* **4**: 250–252.

Dickneite G, Pragst I (2009) Prothrombin complex concentrate vs fresh frozen plasma for reversal of dilutional coagulopathy in a porcine trauma model. *British Journal of Anaesthesia* **102**: 345–354.

Douketis JD, Berger PB, Dunn AS *et al.* (2008) The perioperative management of antithrombotic therapy. American College of Chest Physicians Evidence Based Clinical Practice Guidelines, 8th Edition. *Chest* **133**: 299–339S.

Eisenberg DM, Davis RB, Ettner SL *et al.* (1998) Trends in alternative medicine use in the United States, 1990–1997: results of a follow up national survey. *Journal of the American Medical Association* **280**: 1569–1575.

Evans SJ, Biss TT, Wells RH (2008) Emergency warfarin reversal with prothrombin complex concentrates: United Kingdom wide study. *British Journal of Haematology* **141**: 260–273.

Farooq V, Hegarty J, Chandrasekar T *et al.* (2004) Serious adverse incidents with the usage of low molecular weight heparins in patients with chronic kidney disease. *American Journal of Kidney Disease* **43**: 531–537.

Fernandez MA, Ballesteros S, Aznar J (1998) Oral anticoagulants and insecticides. *Thrombosis and Haemostasis* **80**: 724–726.

Fitzmaurice D, Blann A, Lip GYH (2002) Bleeding risks of antithrombotic therapy. *British Medical Journal* **325**: 828–831.

Gallerani M, Manfredini R, Moratelli S (1995) Non-haemorrhagic adverse reactions of oral anticoagulant therapy. *International Journal of Cardiology* **49**: 1–7.

Gallus AS, Baker RI, Chong BH *et al.* (2000) Consensus guidelines for warfarin therapy. *Medical Journal of Australia* **172**: 600–605.

Graff J, Hentig N, Misselwitz F *et al.* (2007) Effects of the oral direct factor Xa inhibitor Rivaroxaban on platelet induced thrombin generation and prothrombinase activity. *Journal of Clinical Pharmacology* **47**: 1398–1407.

Grant P (2004) Warfarin and cranberry juice: an interaction? *Journal of Heart Valve Disease* **13**: 25–26.

Greenblatt DJ, Von Moltke LL (2005) Interaction of warfarin with drugs, natural substances and foods. *Journal of Clinical Pharmacology* **45**: 127–132.

Greenblatt D (2006) Cranberry juice and warfarin: is there an interaction? *Anticoagulation Forum* **10**: 1–4.

Greenblatt D, Von Moltke LL, Perloff E *et al.* (2006) Interaction of flurbiprofen with cranberry juice, grape juice, tea and fluconazole: *in vitro* and clinical studies. *Clinical Pharmacology and Therapeutics* **79**: 125–133.

Greinacher A, Eckhardt T, Mussmann J *et al.* (1993) Pregnancy complicated by heparin associated thrombocytopenia: management by a prospectively *in vitro* selected heparinoid. *Thrombosis Research* **71**: 123–126.

Greinacher A, Potzsch B, Amiral J *et al.* (1994) Heparin associated thrombocytopenia: isolation of the antibody and characterization of a multimolecular

PF4–heparin complex as the major antigen. *Thrombosis and Haemostasis* **71**: 247–251.

Hirsh J (1998) Low molecular weight heparin: a review of the results of recent studies of the treatment of venous thromboembolism and unstable angina. *Circulation* **98**: 1575–1582.

Hirsh J, Anand SS, Halperin JL *et al.* (2001a) Guide to anticoagulant therapy: heparin. *Circulation* **103**: 2994–3018.

Hirsh J, Dalen JE, Anderson DR *et al.* (2001b) Oral anticoagulants: mechanism of action, clinical effectiveness, and optimal therapeutic range. *Chest* **119**: 8–21S.

Hirsh J, Fuster V, Ansell J *et al.* (2003) American Heart Association/American College of Cardiology foundation guide to warfarin therapy. *Circulation* **107**: 1692–1711.

Hirsh J, Raschke R (2004) Heparin and low molecular weight heparin. *Chest* **126**: 188–203S.

Hirsh J, Bauer KA, Donati MB *et al.* (2008) Parenteral anticoagulants. *Chest* **133**: 141–159S.

Holbrook AM, Pereira JA, Labiris R *et al.* (2005) Systematic overview of warfarin and its drug and food interactions. *Archives of Internal Medicine* **165**: 1095–1106.

Hull R, Hirsh J, Jay R *et al.* (1982) Different intensities of oral anticoagulant therapy in the treatment of proximal vein thrombosis. *New England Journal of Medicine* **307**: 1676–1681.

Hyers TM (2003) Management of venous thromboembolism. *Archives of Internal Medicine* **163**: 759–768.

Hylek E, Singer DE (1994) Risk factors for intracranial hemorrhage in outpatients taking warfarin. *Annals of Internal Medicine* **120**: 897–902.

Izzo AA, Ernst E (2001) Interactions between herbal medicines and prescribed drugs: a systematic review. *Drugs* **61**: 2163–2175.

Jaffer AK, Brotman DJ, Chukwumerije N (2003) When patients on warfarin need surgery. *Cleveland Clinic Journal of Medicine* **70**: 973–984.

Karlson B, Leijd B, Hellstrom K (1986) On the influence of vitamin K rich vegetables and wine on the effectiveness of warfarin treatment. *Acta Medica Scandinavica* **220**: 347–350.

Kearon C, Hirsh J (1997) Management of anticoagulation before and after elective surgery. *New England Journal of Medicine* **336**: 1506–1511.

Kearon C, Kahn SR, Agnelli G *et al.* (2008) Antithrombotic therapy for venous thromboembolic disease. American College of Chest Physicians evidence based clinical practice guidelines, 8th Edition. *Chest* **133**: 454–545.

Kempin SJ (1983) Warfarin resistance caused by broccoli. *New England Journal of Medicine* **308**: 1229–1235.

Landefeld S, Beyth RJ (1993) Anticoagulant related bleeding: clinical epidemiology, prediction and prevention. *American Journal of Medicine* **95**: 315–328.

Laposta MN, Green D, Van Cott EM *et al.* (1998) College of American Pathologists Conference XXXI on laboratory monitoring of anticoagulant therapy: the clinical use and laboratory monitoring of low molecular weight heparin, danaparoid, hirudin and related compounds and argatroban. *Archives of Pathology and Laboratory Medicine* **122**: 799–808.

Levine MN, Raskob G, Landefeld S *et al.* (2001) Hemorrhagic complications of anticoagulant treatment. *Chest* **119**: 108–121S.

Lilja JJ, Backman JT, Neuvonen PJ (2007) Effects of daily ingestion of cranberry juice on the pharmacokinetics of warfarin, tizanidine and midazolam probes of CYP2C9, CYP1A2 and CYP3A4. *Clinical Pharmacology and Therapeutics* **81**: 833–839.

Lim W, Dentali F, Elkelboom JW *et al.* (2006) Meta-analysis: low molecular weight heparin and bleeding in patients with severe renal insufficiency. *Annals of Internal Medicine* **144**: 673–684.

Loeliger EA, van der Besselaar AM, Lewis SM (1985) Reliability and clinical impact of the normalisation of the prothrombin times in oral anticoagulant control. *Thrombosis and Haemostasis* **53**: 148–158.

MacCorquodale DW, Binkley SB, Thayer SA *et al.* (1939) On the constitution of vitamin K1. *Journal of the American Chemical Society* **61**: 1928–1929.

Magnani HN (1993) Heparin induced thrombocytopenia (HIT): an overview of 230 patients treated with orgaran. *Thrombosis and Haemostasis* **70**: 554–561.

Makris M, Greaves M, Phillips WS *et al.* (1997) Emergency oral anticoagulant reversal: the relative efficacy of infusions of fresh frozen plasma and clotting factor concentrate on correction of the coagulopathy. *Thrombosis and Haemostasis* **77**: 477–480.

McLean J (1916) The thromboplastic action of cephalin. *American Journal of Physiology* **41**: 250–257.

Medical Research Council (1998) General Practice Research Framework Thrombosis Prevention Trial: randomised trial of low intensity oral anticoagulation with warfarin and low dose aspirin in the primary prevention of ischaemic heart disease in men at increased risk. *Lancet* **351**: 233–240.

Nijkeuter M, Huisman MV (2004) Pentasaccharides in the prophylaxis and treatment of venous thromboembolism: a systematic review. *Current Opinions in Pulmonary Medicine* **10**: 338–344.

O'Reilly RA, Kearns P (1995) Intravenous vitamin K1 injections: dangerous prophylaxis. *Archives of Internal Medicine* **155**: 2127–2128.

Orme MLE, Lewis PJ, de Swiet M *et al.* (1977) May mothers given warfarin breast feed their children. *British Medical Journal* **1**: 1564–1566.

Overman RS, Stahmann MA, Sullivan WR *et al.* (1941) Studies on the haemorrhagic sweet clover disease. IV. The isolation and crystallization of the haemorrhagic agent. Journal of Biological Chemistry **141**: 941.

Palareti G, Leali N, Coccheri S *et al.* (1996) Bleeding complications of oral anti-coagulant treatment: an inception-cohort prospective collaborative study (ISCOAT). *Lancet* **348**: 423–428.

Pell JP, McIver B, Stuart P *et al.* (1993) Comparison of anticoagulant control among patients attending general practice and a hospital anticoagulant clinic. *British Journal of General Practice* **43**: 152–157.

Poller L, Shiach CR, MacCallum PK *et al.* (1998) Multicentre randomised study of computerised anticoaulant dosage. *Lancet* **352**: 1505–1509.

Ramstrom G, Sindet-Pedersen S, Hall G *et al.* (1993) Prevention of postsurgical bleeding in oral surgery using tranexamic acid without dose modification of oral anticoagulants. *Journal of Oral and Maxillofacial Surgery* **54**: 27–34.

Raschke RA, Gollihare B, Peirce JC (1996) The effectiveness of implementing the weight based heparin nomogram as a practice guideline. *Archives of Internal Medicine* **156**: 1645–1649.

Raskob GE, Hull RD, Pineo GF (2001) Heparin, hirudin and related agents. In Beutler E, Lichtman MA, Coller BS *et al.* (eds), *Williams' Hematology*, 6th Edition. McGraw-Hill, New York: 1793–1801.

Rindone J, Murphy T (2006) Warfarin–cranberry juice interaction resulting in profound hypoprothrombinemia and bleeding. *American Journal of Therapeutics* **13**: 283–284.

Sallah S, Thomas DP, Roberts HR (1997) Warfarin and heparin induced skin necrosis and the purple toe syndrome: infrequent complications of anticoagulant treatment. *Thrombosis and Haemostasis* **78**: 785–789.

Sanson BJ, Lensing AWA, Prins MH *et al.* (1999) Safety of low molecular weight heparin in pregnancy: a systematic review. *Thrombosis and Haemostasis* **81**: 668–672.

Stein PD, Alpert JS, Bussey HI *et al.* (2001) Antithrombotic therapy in patients with mechanical and biological prosthetic heart valves. *Chest* **119**: 220–227S [published correction appears in *Chest* **120**: 1044].

Schofield FW (1922) A brief account of a disease in cattle simulating hemorrhagic septicaemia due to feeding sweet clover. *Canadian Veterinary Record* **3**: 74.

Schulman S (2001) Oral anticoagulation. In Beutler E, Lichtman MA, Coller BS *et al.* (eds), *Williams' Hematology*, 6th Edition. McGraw-Hill, New York: 1777–1792.

Schulman S (2003). Care of patients receiving long-term anticoagulant therapy. *New England Journal of Medicine* **349**: 675–683.

Scully M (2002) Warfarin therapy. Rat poison and the prevention of thrombosis. *Biochemist* **24**: 15–17.

Stevenson RE, Burton OM, Ferlauto GJ *et al.* (1980) Hazards of oral anticoagulants during pregnancy. *Journal of the American Medical Association* **243**: 1549–1555.

Sullivan DM, Ford MA, Boyden TW (1998) Grapefruit juice and the response to warfarin. *American Journal of Health System Pharmacy* **55**: 1581–1583.

Suvarna R, Pirmohamed M, Henderson L (2003) Possible interaction between warfarin and cranberry juice. *British Medical Journal* **327**: 1454.

Tatsumi A, Kadobayashi M (2007) Effect of alcohol on the binding of warfarin enantiomers to human serum albumin. *BioPharm Bulletin* **30**: 826–829.

Thorevska N, Amoateng-Adjepong Y, Sabahi R *et al.* (2004) Anticoagulation in hospitalized patients with renal insufficiency. A comparison of bleeding rates with unfractionated heparin vs enoxaparin. *Chest* **125**: 856–863.

Turpie AGG, Gallus AS, Hoek JA (2001) A synthetic pentasaccharide for the prevention of deep vein thrombosis after total hip replacement. *New England Journal of Medicine* **344**: 619–625.

Van der Meer FJM, Rosendaal FR, Vandenbroucke JP *et al.* (1993) Bleeding complications in oral anticoagulant therapy: an analysis of risk factors. *Archives of Internal Medicine* **153**: 1557–1562.

Warkentin TE, Kelton JG (1996) A 14 year study of heparin induced thrombocytopenia. *American Journal of Medicine* **101**: 505–510.

Warkentin TE, Greinacher A (2004) Heparin induced thrombocytopenia: recognition, treatment and prevention. *Chest* **126**: 311–337S.

Weitz JI, Hirsh J, Samama MM. (2004) New anticoagulant drugs. *Chest* **126**: 265–286S.

Whitling AM, Bussey BI, Lyons RM (1998) Comparing different routes and doses of phytonadione for reversing excessive anticoagulation. *Archives of Internal Medicine* **158**: 2136–2140.

Wittkowsky AK, Bussey HI, Walker MB *et al.* (2007) Dietary supplement use among anticoagulation clinic patients. *Journal of Thrombosis and Haemostasis* **5**: 875–877.

Wittkowsky AK (2008) Dietary supplements, herbs and oral anticoagulants: the nature of the evidence. *Journal of Thrombosis and Thrombolysis* **25**: 72–77.

Wood MJ, Stewart RL, Merry H *et al.* (2003) Use of complementary and alternative medical therapies in patients with cardiovascular disease. *American Heart Journal* **145**: 806–812.

Yeager BF, Matheny SC (1999) Low molecular weight heparin in outpatient treatment of DVT. American Family Physician. Available at: www.aafp. org/afp/99021ap/945.html

Zhaoping LI, Seerman NP, Carpenter CL *et al.* (2006) Cranberry does not affect prothrombin time in male subjects on warfarin. *Journal of the American Dietetic Association* **106**: 2057–2061.

Nursing interventions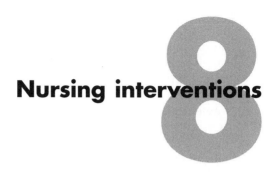

Nurses are at the centre of a national strategy to reduce deaths from VTE.

(Chief Nursing Officer, 2009)

Overview

This statement by the Chief Nursing Officer acknowledges the importance of the nurse's role in implementing both evidence-based VTE risk assessment tools to assess hospitalized patients' individual risk of VTE, combined with evidence-based thrombo-prophylaxis, such as anti-embolism stockings (AES), intermittent pneumatic compression (IPC), foot pumps, electrical stimulation devices and anticoagulation.

Successful implementation of VTE risk assessment and thromboprophylaxis requires strong leadership and project management skills. Leadership skills are often assumed to be achievable without specific preparation (Wright 1996). This assumption is also often applied to project management skills, in which nurses are not usually formally taught, and yet implementation is a core part of the nursing process.

Venous Thromboembolism: A Nurses Guide to Prevention and Management   By Ellen Welch
© 2010 John Wiley & Sons, Ltd.

This chapter will focus on two main areas:

1. Thromboprophylaxis with AES, IPC, foot pumps and electrical stimulation devices, including physiology, contraindications, application, nursing care and evidence base, and practical administration of LMWH injections.
2. Implementation, including practical application of leadership and project management skills and tools, the nurse's role in the procurement of evidence-based products and informing the patient.

Practical thromboprophylaxis

As previously discussed in earlier chapters, the aim of thromboprophylaxis is to prevent VTE by targeting Virchow's triad of predisposing factors: venous stasis, vein wall trauma or dilatation and hypercoagulability (Virchow 1856) (Figure 8.1). Logic suggests that the more components of the triad that are targeted by thromboprophylaxis, the lower the risk of VTE.

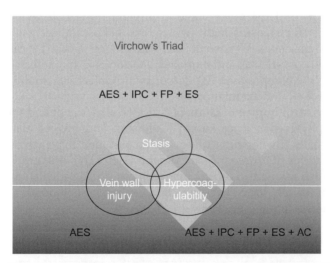

Figure 8.1 Virchow's triad. AC, Anticoagulants; AES, anti-embolism stocking; IPC, intermittent pneumatic compression; FP, foot pump; ES, electrical stimulation.

Anti-embolism stockings

Physiology

AES provide continuous stimulation of linear blood flow, prevent venous dilatation (Coleridge Smith *et al.* 1991) and stimulate endothelial fibrinolytic activity (Arcelus *et al.* 1995). Thigh-length stockings offer increased protection above the knee, compared with knee-length stockings, by increasing blood flow velocity in the femoral vein and preventing dilatation of the popliteal vein (Benko *et al.* 1999).

Contraindications

Contraindications to the use of AES include:

- Local leg conditions.
- Arteriosclerosis or other ischaemic vascular disease or diabetic neuropathy.
- Massive oedema of legs or pulmonary oedema from congestive heart failure.
- Extreme deformity of the legs.
- Patient refusal to wear the stockings correctly.

Application and nursing care

Anyone applying AES should have received training on indications, contraindications, how to measure the patient's legs, how to select the appropriate-sized stocking based on the patient's measurements, how to apply the stockings and where to place the thigh gusset.

Before AES can be used, the patient must be measured to select the right style and size of stockings, which can be done with the patient either in bed or standing up, and the measurements recorded on the patient's notes. First, the circumference of the thigh is measured at the widest point, to determine whether or not the patient can be safely fitted into the thigh-length style (from the stocking manufacturer's upper limit) or will need either a thigh-length stocking with belt or a knee-length stocking.

Next, the circumference of the calf is measured at the widest point, with both calves measured if there is an obvious difference in size. It may be necessary to fit two different sizes of stockings. Finally, to determine the length of leg, the distance from the gluteal furrow (buttock fold) to the heel is measured if fitting the patient for a thigh-length or thigh-length with belt style; or from the popliteal fold (bend behind the knee) to the heel if a knee-length style is to be used. The manufacturer's fitting guide is used to select the appropriate size of stocking, based on the three measurements obtained. The size chosen and applied should be documented in the patient's notes. This process may need to be repeated if a patient's legs become more or less swollen, depending on their underlying medical condition.

Figure 8.2 shows how the stockings are fitted.

Clinicians should monitor the use of the stockings by checking the circulation (warmth, colour, sensation) via the toe hole in the stocking. The patient should be advised to report any numbness or tingling while wearing the stockings, which should be removed daily for washing (follow the manufacturer's instructions) and to check that the patient's skin is intact. Supplying two pairs of stockings will allow for one pair to be washed and dried whilst the other pair is worn, as it is advisable for them to be left off for no longer than 30 minutes. Both verbal and written information on the stockings should be given to the patient. Some patients may have difficulty in applying the stockings and may need assistance to put them on.

Evidence base

NICE (2007) advise that patients should be encouraged to wear their stockings from admission until they return to their usual levels of mobility, and that staff should 'inform them that this will reduce their risk of VTE'. However, it is not necessary to demonstrate that a mechanical thromboprophylaxis device provides any protection against VTE in order for it to be approved and marketed (Geerts *et al.* 2008). Although many of these devices have never been assessed in any clinical trial, there is an unsubstantiated assumption that they are all effective and equivalent (Geerts *et al.* 2008). The NMC Code of Conduct (2008) states that 'You must ensure any advice you give is evidence based if you are suggesting healthcare products or services'.

To adhere to the Code of Conduct (2008) and the NICE (2007) recommendations, and in light of the ACCP (Geerts *et al.* 2008) comments, it

---

▶

Figure 8.2 Fitting anti-embolism stockings. (a) To fit the stockings on the patient, put your hand inside the stocking and grasp the heel (this is usually visible in some way, such as a change in the stitching pattern). While holding onto the heel, pull the stocking inside out. There are devices available on the market that can assist with application (please see manufacturer's instructions if using these).

(b) Place the stocking over the foot, ensuring the heel is placed in the heel pocket. The toe hole should be placed under the toes. It is important that patients do not leave their toes out through the toe hole as this may cause pressure damage to the skin.

(c) Grasp the top of the stocking and pull it back over the heel and up the leg. Smooth the stocking to ensure there are no wrinkles that could cause skin damage.

(d) Ensure the thigh gusset is adjusted to fit over the inside of the thigh. Early work by Sigel stressed the importance of having a gusset instead of a continuous band at the top of the stocking, to prevent constriction over the femoral vein.

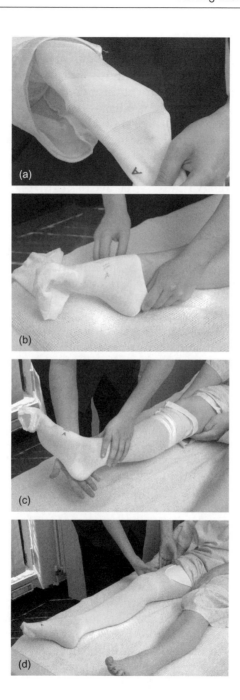

becomes increasingly evident that clinicians need to start questioning the clinical evidence behind the VTE thromboprophylaxis products being used in their organization, and work collaboratively with their Procurement Departments, Thrombosis Committee and budget holders to ensure that evidence-based products are used.

For their evidence-based review of AES, NICE (2007) selected nine randomized controlled trials that had DVT diagnosis as the endpoint. Of the 693 patients in the AES group and 651 in the no-stocking control group, 88 and 158 patients, respectively, suffered a DVT. Thus, AES reduced the risk of DVT by 53% [relative risk (RR) 0.47, 95% confidence interval (CI) 0.32–0.69) (NICE, 2007).

To try to classify AES, NICE (2007) recommended that AES should provide compression equivalent to Sigel's (1975) profile (a pressure profile for elastic stockings). Unfortunately, as many AES are currently manufactured to meet the British Standard (BS) for AES 7672 (1993), and as there are several areas where the current British Standard for AES does not correspond to Sigel's profile, the BS needs to be amended if it is to be useful as a standard of safety of a product. However, clinicians should be aware that a BS does not endorse the effectiveness of a product. Not all manufacturers have adhered to the BS, which was developed in 1993, several years after much of the research into the effectiveness of AES had already been done, and therefore, understandably, their products have remained unchanged and still have valid research. However, if the BS is updated and AES are modified to meet it, then research conducted on the product's effectiveness prior to the modification will be invalidated – and not all manufacturers will choose to adhere to an updated BS for AES. Clinicians should keep abreast of developments in this area and review their choice of AES critically.

It is unfortunately not sufficient to extrapolate research from one brand of stocking to another and assume it will be just as effective, because of numerous variations in manufacturing techniques, materials used, the way fabric is knitted, fabric stiffness, size ranges available, presence or not of a thigh gusset or popliteal break and differences in National and International standards for manufacture. It would be unacceptable to extrapolate research from one brand of LMWH to another, yet it has been practice to do this with AES over many years and manufacturers often justify the lack of research on their product as expensive and difficult to carry out. Clinicians should challenge this view and, along with the industry, facilitate ethically approved randomized controlled trials to enhance the evidence base behind the use of AES, particularly in medical patients where there is a dearth of research.

Often clinicians are approached to conduct 'comfort' trials (trials where one white stocking is compared against another, to see which one the patient prefers to wear, based on the comfort of the fabric). If proceeding with this, ethical approval needs to be sought first, to ensure that patients are not put at risk if comparing a proven product to one that is unproven.

Clinicians have debated which length of stocking (knee- or thigh-length) is best over the years, but evidence-based practice and national guidance have supported the use of thigh-length stockings (SIGN 2002; NICE 2007). Although clinicians still debate the 'ideal compression profile' and which machine or standard it should be measured against, evidence-based practice supports the use of a product that has demonstrated an ability to reduce DVT incidence. A simple way of reviewing the research on a product is to review which products were used in the studies included in either AES meta-analyses or studies from which national guidelines were formed. As long as the product has shown a statistically significant reduction in DVT rates and is still manufactured to the same criteria, then it could be considered to be evidence-based.

Intermittent pneumatic compression (IPC; leg sleeves)

Physiology
IPC empties blood from behind the valve cusps, preventing venous stasis and increasing blood flow velocity. The following studies support the ability of IPC to enhance fibrinolysis. A twofold increase in tissue factor pathway inhibitor antigen levels was observed in volunteers wearing long-leg IPC sleeves for 1 hour (Hoppensteadt et al. 1995). Temporary venous occlusion (such as occurs with cyclic sequential compression) in the lower limb is thought to stimulate the venous endothelium to release tissue plasminogen activator (Hartmann 1982). IPC applied to the leg induces significant increases in fibrin and fibrinogen degradation products (short-lived), so IPC is only effective while it is applied, therefore non-contiguous use of IPC may result in suboptimal thromboprophylaxis (Jacobs et al. 1996).

Contraindications
IPC must not be applied if the patient has a DVT (or suspected DVT), as it may increase the risk of embolization. Other contraindications are the same as those for AES.

Application and nursing care
Figure 8.3 shows how IPC is fitted. IPC or foot impulse devices can be used as alternatives to, or in addition to, graduated compression

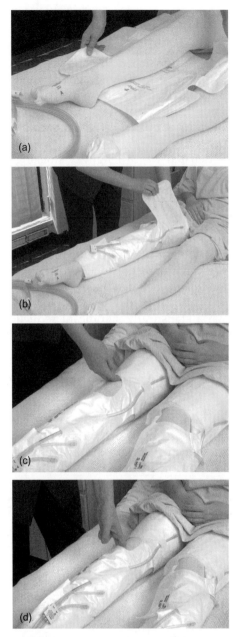

Figure 8.3 Fitting intermittent pneumatic compression (IPC).

(a) To fit the leggings, place the legging flat underneath the patient's leg. The legging is marked to show which way round it should be applied to ensure the popliteal break is in the correct position.

(b) Wrap the leggings snugly around the calf and thigh.

(c, d) Using two fingers, check that they can slip easily underneath the leggings, both above and below the knee. This ensures that they are not wrapped too tightly around the patient's legs.

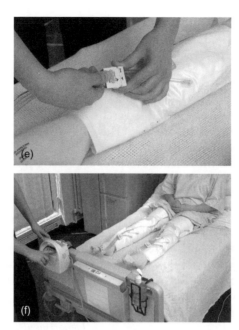

Figure 8.3 (*Continued*) (e) Connect the tubing on the legging to the tubing on the controller by pushing until it snaps into place.
(f) Advise the patient that he/she can detach him/herself from the tubing if there is a need to move from the bed. Follow the manufacturer's instructions when operating the controller.

stockings (GCS) while patients are in hospital (NICE, 2007). If used on the ward, IPC or foot impulse devices should be worn for as much of the time as is practical while the patient is in bed or sitting on a chair.

If the device has been switched off for a prolonged period, the patient should be cautiously reassessed for signs of acute DVT prior to reapplying the device. It is important to check and document the circulation in the patient's feet shortly after application of IPC devices.

As for all the mechanical methods of thromboprophylaxis, the patient should be advised to report immediately any new symptoms, such as numbness, tingling, colour changes or discomfort in their feet or legs. They should also be advised to report any symptoms of VTE, such as leg pain or swelling, or chest symptoms such as shortness of breath, chest pains or haemoptysis.

Evidence base
Urbankova *et al.* (2005) assessed the effectiveness of IPC in preventing DVT in postoperative patients in a meta-analysis of 15 studies. Of 2270

patients, 1125 were fitted with IPC and 1145 received no thrombo-prophylaxis. IPC reduced the risk of DVT by 60% compared with no thromboprophylaxis (RR, 0.40; 95% CI, 0.29–0.56; $p < 0.001$)

Foot pumps

Foot pumps are a form of IPC whereby a foot cuff is attached to the controller instead of leg sleeves. They have been given their own section in this chapter, as the physiology, contraindications, application and evidence base differ from those for IPC using leg sleeves.

Physiology
The sole of the foot contains a plexus of veins, the venae comitantes of the lateral plantar artery, and normal weight bearing expels blood from this plexus, causing a pulse of blood to pass through the deep veins of the lower leg, which reduces venous stasis and liberates fibrinolytic factors from the venous endothelial wall. The foot-pump system reproduces the rhythmic expression of blood from the plexus when a patient cannot bear weight

(Department of Health 2007)

Contraindications
Foot pumps are contraindicated in patients with conditions where an increase of fluid to the heart may be detrimental, such as congestive heart failure, or with pre-existing DVT, thrombophlebitis or PE. Caution should be used when fitting foot pumps for patients with an infected or insensitive extremity.

Application
The foot cuffs are applied to the feet and attached to a controller similar to that used for IPC leg sleeves. Often foot-pumps are used instead of IPC when access to the patient's leg is difficult, for example, if they have external fixations to their legs (see Figure 8.4).

Evidence base
IPC has been compared with foot pumps in 149 patients after non-lower extremity trauma. DVTs were found by ultrasound in four of 62 patients fitted with IPC and 13 of 62 fitted with foot pumps (6.5% versus 21%; $p = 0.009$). All four DVTs in the IPC group were unilateral, while seven in the foot-pump group were bilateral (Elliott *et al.* 1999). This suggests that IPC is more effective than foot-pumps; however, further research is needed to confirm this.

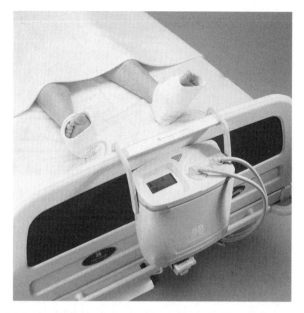

Figure 8.4 Picture of foot pump being worn. Reproduced with permission. © Arjo-Huntleigh group of companies 2009.

Electrical stimulation devices

Physiology
Electrical stimulation-induced contractions have been shown to activate the skeletal muscle pump and promote limb blood flow velocity (Faghri *et al.* 1997).

Contraindications
Electrical stimulation devices should not be used in patients with cardiac pacemakers or in pregnant women. Gel electrodes should not be applied over an open wound and stimulation should not be applied:

- To any part of the body other than the calf muscle.
- To a patient who is not fully anaesthetized (may not be applicable to newer devices).
- When clinical signs and symptoms of venous occlusion are present.
- Over or in close proximity to cancerous lesions.

Application
Electrical stimulation devices are currently applied only on unconscious patients in theatre. Straps are placed around the patient's calf and the device works from a battery source (see Figure 8.5).

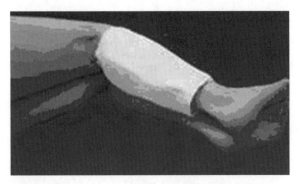

Figure 8.5 Picture of electrical stimulation device being worn. Picture supplied by AMTEC Consulting plc.

Evidence base

Favourable results have been shown when electrical stimulation is used on its own or with IPC and AES, but only very small numbers of patients were included in the studies (NICE 2007). Newer painless devices targeted at the popliteal nerve are currently being developed and may become the future of mechanical thromboprophylaxis, once clinical trials support their efficacy in reducing the incidence of DVT.

Anticoagulants

Drugs such as LMWH reduce hypercoagulability by inhibiting coagulation proteins through increased antithrombin action, and are discussed further in Chapter 7. New oral anticoagulants such as dabigatran and rivaroxaban are now available, targeting coagulation factors such as factor IIa (thrombin) and factor Xa.

Patients may be required to self-administer heparin as treatment for VTE as an outpatient or for continuing thromboprophylaxis when discharged from hospital. It is often feasible for patients to administer LMWH, but individuals should be assessed to ensure they have sufficient mental and physical capacity to perform the task and are likely to adhere to treatment. Written and verbal information as well as a contact number for queries or problems should be given, and patients should be assessed as they practise injection technique, ideally on a dummy. Patients should be observed self-injecting on at least one occasion to ensure competence, and their competence should be documented. General medication advice should be given to patients, such as storage, timing, expiry dates and procedures, in case of accidental overdose or missed doses.

How to teach a patient to self-administer LMWH

This is demonstrated in Figure 8.6.

The patient should dispose of the syringe safely and store the sharps bin out of reach of children. These stages can be practised until the patient feels comfortable. Self-injection should then be observed to ensure competence and encourage adherence.

The design of the injection (needle and syringe) may differ. Some may have a retractable needle or have a safety feature to reduce the chance of needle stick injury. Follow the manufacturer's advice regarding their administration.

If the patient is unable to self-administer, then relatives or district nurses may be involved at this point to assist with administration.

Implementation

Leadership for implementation

Minimizing the risk of VTE for all hospitalized patients through VTE risk assessment and thromboprophylaxis involves a change in the culture or practice for many organizations. The leadership required to facilitate this change needs to balance the vision with the reality of the resources available, and leaders need to have the courage and motivation to take ownership of the vision to improve the chances of successful implementation. This requires a range of leadership skills and knowledge, such as negotiation skills, conflict management, organizational culture, power and influence and an awareness of one's own leadership style. *Shifting the Balance of Power* (DH 2002), a Department of Health publication, reinforced the importance of nursing leadership as a catalyst for change. Being prepared for a leadership challenge such as this involves gaining an academic knowledge of leadership, combined with previous experience, in order to influence colleagues to complete VTE risk assessment forms and deliver thromboprophylaxis for all patients.

The decision as to who should perform VTE risk assessment should be made locally and may differ depending on the local culture of each individual ward. The culture in most organizations is that nurses carry out risk assessments (such as for falls), and deliver thromboprophylaxis, therefore they may be best placed to conduct VTE risk assessment. Pre-assessment nurses are in an ideal position to perform VTE risk assessment for elective surgical patients. However, on a medical ward it may be more appropriate for the doctor to conduct VTE risk assessment as part of the admission process and prescribe the thromboprophylaxis for the nurse to administer. In most areas the nurses will

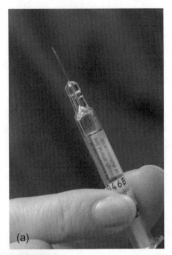

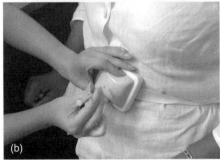

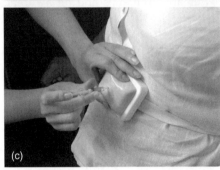

Figure 8.6 Teaching a patient how to self-inject low molecular weight heparin (LMWH). (a) Explain the injection technique to the patient. Demonstrate removal of the cap by pulling it off firmly. Advise the patient not to twist the cap to avoid damage to the needle. Explain that air should not be expelled from the syringe.

(b) Demonstrate injection administration to the patient on a simulation abdomen. Gently pinch an area at least 5 cm from the umbilicus on either side of the abdomen to make a fold in the skin. Insert the needle at 90 degrees into the skin fold. Ensure that the full length of the needle is inserted.

(c) Press the plunger all the way down with your finger. Remove the needle by pulling it out at 90 degrees and let go of the skin.

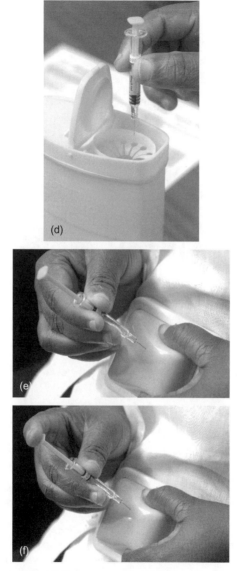

Figure 8.6 (*Continued*) (d) Demonstrate and explain safe disposal of the syringe. Advise the patient what to do with the bin when it's full.

(e, f) Instruct the patient to practise the technique him/herself while talking through each stage. Advise the patient to hold the syringe in his/her dominant hand and gently pinch an area on the simulation abdomen with the other hand to make a skin fold. Instruct the patient to insert the needle into the skin fold, observing to ensure that it is inserted at 90 degrees.

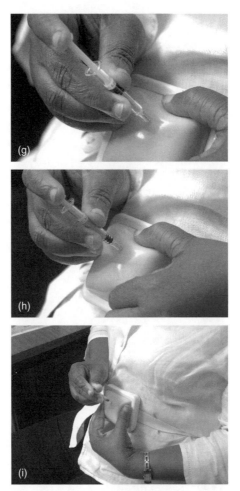

Figure 8.6 (*Continued*) (g) The patient should insert the full length of the needle into the skin at a rate he/she feels comfortable with. Advise the patient to push the plunger down steadily with his/her finger.

(h) Ensure that the patient administers all of the injection.

(i) Observe the patient removing the needle at 90 degrees from the abdomen and advise him/her to release the skin fold. Warn the patient against rubbing the area to avoid excessive bruising.

be at the front line of thromboprophylaxis delivery. The nurse's approach to minimizing the risk of VTE may be best implemented through the nursing process of assessing, planning, implementing and evaluating the needs of individual patients through the development of a 'nursing care plan' (see Box 8.1), as is the usual practice or culture

Box 8.1 Nursing care plan for a patient at risk of venous thromboembolism (VTE)

Problem

Mrs patient X is potentially at risk of VTE due to hospitalization.

Goal

To minimize her risk of VTE.

Nursing interventions

- Provide verbal and written information regarding risk of VTE and thromboprophylaxis.
- Assess risk using VTE risk assessment tool or ensure doctor has completed the risk assessment.
- Ensure risk assessment outcome has been documented in patient records.
- Document which thromboprophylaxis modalities are appropriate, depending on the level of risk.
- Check and record whether there are any contraindications to thromboprophylaxis.
- Ensure that thromboprophylaxis is prescribed on the patient's drug chart.
- Administer or apply thromboprophylaxis as per drug chart.
- Measure and document size of the patient's foot/calf/thigh/ length of leg, as appropriate, depending on which thromboprophylaxis modality is used, and size of stocking/sleeve or foot cuff applied, and follow manufacturer's instructions regarding washing.
- Consider the patient's cultural and spiritual beliefs and gain consent prior to administering LMWH, as it is porcine-derived, or seek alternative from doctor.
- Encourage mobilization (if medically fit) and leg and deep breathing exercises (refer to physiotherapist if necessary).
- Make clinical observations 4–6 hourly (blood pressure, pulse, respirations) and observe her legs for signs of DVT.
- Check for side-effects of thromboprophylaxis and report immediately to doctor (including checking skin integrity and circulation).
- Inform the patient that she should watch for signs and symptoms of VTE or adverse effects from thromboprophylaxis and report them to a clinician immediately.

- If the patient's VTE risk factors change, ensure that her risk is reassessed as soon as possible.
- Document date and time when mechanical thromboprophylaxis is removed.
- Ensure that the patient's VTE risk on discharge is considered and decide whether or not thromboprophylaxis needs to be continued and, if so, for how long.
- Other ....

Evaluation date: ....

when identifying and caring for patient needs. The care plan needs to have regular evaluations as the patient's VTE risk factors may change.

The nurse's choice of leadership style is relevant. For prevention of VTE, which requires a high level of commitment from healthcare workers to ensure effective risk assessment and thromboprophylaxis provision, a transformational leadership style is preferred – engaging with and empowering colleagues in such a way that those involved are raised to higher levels of motivation and morality (Burns 1978). An educational presentation on morbidity and mortality of VTE, showing the value of reducing the risk for patients by completing the risk assessment forms, followed by a series of face-to-face meetings (to facilitate negotiation and manage potential conflict), will ensure that nurses are more likely to accept this change to their role, perceiving the change as legitimate (an important power source) and ensuring a shared vision, therefore promoting the chance of successful implementation.

Procurement

If nurses are to believe in the value of the mechanical thromboprophylaxis they are administering, they need to be confident that the products are evidence-based. Appropriate procurement requires selecting and supplying a quality (evidence-based) product and nurses need to have a leading role in the selection process. This can be a daunting and time-consuming task for nurses and requires critical analysis of the research available on the particular product, along with leadership skills to assist with the decision-making process.

In an effort to ease the difficulties healthcare professionals face when choosing AES and to provide impartial and objective information, a compression hosiery buyer's guide was developed by the Centre for Evidence-based Purchasing (CEP), which was established as part of the Purchasing and Supply Agency (CEP 2008). This guide looks at various

---

Box 8.2 Practical decision making for procurement of AES at King's College Hospital NHS Foundation Trust

In the King's College Hospital NSH Foundation Trust, the Thrombosis Committee led the review and evaluation of AES and chose a cost-effective brand of stocking for which there was clinical evidence of its ability to reduce the incidence of DVT, thereby reducing the costs of treating DVT/PE/post-thrombotic syndrome and reducing the possible costs of litigation. The evidence was obtained from studies eligible for inclusion in the guidance from Amarigiri *et al.* (2003), the Scottish Intercollegiate Guidance Network (SIGN 2002) and NICE (2007). Once this selection process was documented and agreement on the product obtained, the information was fed back to the MSSG and standardization of the product was rolled out across the Trust. Other products were 'masked', meaning that clinicians were unable to order other AES products unless specifically negotiated with procurement. Industry facilitated the change by ensuring that staff were trained and that tape measures and literature were available.

---

aspects that will assist clinicians in their decision-making. It includes a template for how to review products and implement the chosen product(s) across the organization, citing the King's College Hospital NHS Foundation Trust model (see Box 8.2 for a practical example):

- The Medical Supplies and Strategy Group (MSSG) reviews products for standardization in the Trust.
- Meetings are chaired by a procurement manager.
- Each directorate nominates a clinician to attend 3-monthly meetings.
- Representatives from specialist disciplines also attend (e.g. infection control nurse, tissue viability nurse, equipment library manager).
- Products are nominated for review, either by clinicians or procurement, and then reviewed and evaluated by 'appropriate clinicians' and the findings are presented to the MSSG for agreement on standardization, based on cost-effectiveness.

Project management for implementation

Practical implementation of a change project requires project management skills. Loo (2003) suggests that project management follows a life cycle from a conceptual phase, through a detailed project planning phase and an implementation phase, to a project termination

---

Box 8.3 Background for project management of IPC implementation

IPC is only effective whilst it is applied to the patient (Jacobs *et al.* 1996) and the risk of VTE persists for the first couple of weeks following surgery (Geerts *et al.* 2008). From my previous experience in visiting our own theatres and other hospitals nationally, these devices are commonly removed when the patient leaves theatre. This means that the patient does not get the maximum benefit of IPC, whereby it should be left *in situ* until he/she is ambulant, at which time the risk of VTE is considered to be reduced and IPC can be removed (Geerts *et al.* 2008). I had met with various stakeholders to agree supply and funding of IPC devices, but not the disposables, and I had already introduced IPC into recovery and onto one of the six surgical wards in our trust.

---

phase. The following reviews practical project management tools and uses the implementation of IPC on surgical wards as an example (see Box 8.3).

Conceptual phase

Situational analysis (SA) and its questioning nature is useful to establish the scope of the problem and prioritize it to enable strategic planning of the overall service. It is similar to a strengths, weaknesses, opportunities and threats (SWOT) analysis (see Box 8.4), which can help the Project Manager to decide whether or not to pursue the proposed project, as weaknesses and threats may heavily outweigh strengths and opportunities, making the chances of the project succeeding small – therefore time may be better spent elsewhere (Loo 2003). Project description (see Box 8.5) is an important communication tool for the project team, management and other stakeholders (Loo R 2003). It should give a concise overview of the project and is particularly useful to have when presenting the project to others.

Project planning phase

Newton (2005) advocates the need to analyse what the planning is for and who the target audience is, and adapt the plan accordingly. The Project Manager is accountable for the end result, so should ensure that everyone's role is incorporated into the project plan (Newton 2005).

Box 8.4 SWOT analysis

Strengths
- Project aim has strong evidence base
- Exemplar status put us in strong negotiating position for funding
- Backing of Chief Executive and management
- Willingness of staff, internal and external, to provide training who have excellent communication/ presentation skills
- Knowledge of the organizational culture and structure
- Much of the groundwork already done, including pilot of IPC on ward and introduction of IPC to recovery

Weaknesses
- Relying on trainers to find the time to provide training
- Managers need to allow staff time off the ward to be trained
- Project Manager has little experience of using structured project management tools
- This project is only one part of the Project Manager's overall role within coagulation services and she will not be be able to concentrate solely on this project

Opportunities
- To disseminate experience, nationally enhancing our exemplar status
- To develop project management skills within the manager and team
- To use experience of this project to facilitate future project management
- To conduct research on the impact of IPC in reducing incidence of VTE by using evidence-based practice

Threats
- Staff sickness in a small team would result in the Project Manager having to cover other services and the project may have to be put on hold
- Funding for potential increase in cost for disposables may not be agreed by budget holders
- May not achieve 50% of staff trained on IPC prior to introduction of equipment onto the wards, which would delay project completion

The SWOT analysis provided encouragement that the project aim is still viable. Contingency plans can be developed to tackle the weakness and threats.

Box 8.5 Project description

Project title

Intermittent Pneumatic Compression (IPC).

Unit

Thrombosis Committee Leading Project.

Purpose

To make IPC available for use on the surgical wards, establishing a rolling programme of training in their use.

Terms of reference

- *Project manager:* Coagulation nurse specialist.
- *Project team:* Thrombosis Committee, industry, surgical ward sisters, link nurses, coagulation nurse specialists, Procurement, Medical Engineering Department.
- *Reporting structure:* Project team members to feedback directly to Project Manager once weekly on Wednesday. Weekly updates reported at Thrombosis Committee meeting on Thursday and then disseminated by e-mail to relevant parties.
- *Budget:* Funding for one coagulation nurse specialist secured for 2 years from November 2007. Extended usage of IPC onto the wards may result in increase cost for disposables. Local, national and international guidelines to supporting evidence base.

Methodology and milestones

- Use the following project management tools: situational analysis; SWOT analysis; work breakdown structure; Gantt charts; issues impact assessment worksheet; project status reports.
- Each objective achieved on the due date will be a milestone.
- Project commenced November 2007.
- Project to be completed by 31 January 2009 to coincide with Trust's official launch of an updated VTE risk assessment for surgical patients, as IPC is part of the thromboprophylaxis that may be prescribed.

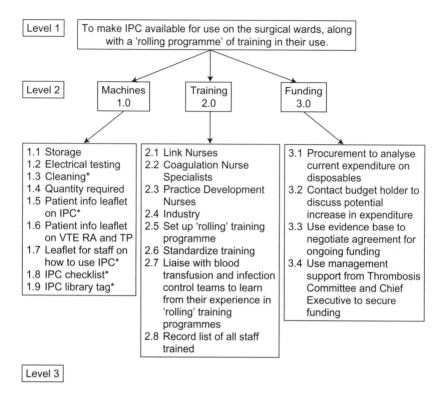

| Level 1 | To make IPC available for use on the surgical wards, along with a 'rolling programme' of training in their use. |

Level 2 — Machines 1.0 | Training 2.0 | Funding 3.0

| Level 3 |

Machines 1.0
1.1 Storage
1.2 Electrical testing
1.3 Cleaning*
1.4 Quantity required
1.5 Patient info leaflet on IPC*
1.6 Patient info leaflet on VTE RA and TP
1.7 Leaflet for staff on how to use IPC*
1.8 IPC checklist*
1.9 IPC library tag*

Training 2.0
2.1 Link Nurses
2.2 Coagulation Nurse Specialists
2.3 Practice Development Nurses
2.4 Industry
2.5 Set up 'rolling' training programme
2.6 Standardize training
2.7 Liaise with blood transfusion and infection control teams to learn from their experience in 'rolling' training programmes
2.8 Record list of all staff trained

Funding 3.0
3.1 Procurement to analyse current expenditure on disposables
3.2 Contact budget holder to discuss potential increase in expenditure
3.3 Use evidence base to negotiate agreement for ongoing funding
3.4 Use management support from Thrombosis Committee and Chief Executive to secure funding

*means task completed

Figure 8.7 Work breakdown structure. The WBS is a graphical tool that displays the project's statement of work, making it easier to understand and communicate. It is employed from the earliest stages of project planning. *Task completed. Loo (2003).

A work breakdown structure (WBS) is a planning tool that uses the key assumption that the Project Manager must start with the end in mind (Shirey 2008). Billows (2008) suggests using the question, 'What work needs to be done to accomplish the objectives?'. The work breakdown structure (WBS; see Figure 8.7) can facilitate the formation of specific, measurable, achievable, relevant and time-framed (SMART) objectives (Ambler 2006) (see Box 8.6) and provides a structure from which to form a generic project-planning chart (Loo 2003) (see Table 8.1). This illustrates who is accountable for individual tasks within the project and allows for the estimated time of the tasks to be calculated, along with how much time must elapse before the task can be started within the context of the project.

Contingency planning ensures that the unforeseen is anticipated and appropriate actions are planned, so that the success of the project

---

Box 8.6 SMART objectives

From the WBS there are three specific areas for action, documented in Level 2 (1.0 IPC machines, 2.0 training, 3.0 funding), that are necessary to meet the project aim. SMART objectives can be developed around these:

- A predetermined number of safety checked IPC machines, with all necessary literature, will be stored on the specified ward and available for use on surgical patients throughout the six surgical wards by 31 January 2009.
- A standardized roster of training will be available by designated trainers at predetermined regular intervals and a list of staff trained will be kept by 8 January 2009, with 50% trained by 31 January 2009.
- The surgical budget holder, or other source, will agree funding for any increased cost in disposables by 15 January 2009.

---

is not jeopardized (Loo 2003). An issues analysis chart (see Table 8.2) can be used to determine where extra steps in the project can be taken to address any potential problems.

Implementation phase
Pischke-Winn *et al.* (1996) advise that sources of resistance should be explored and addressed early. It is important not to allow the project to slip behind or fail to take action to deal with difficulties and delays (Haynes 1989). The 'worksheet progress report' (Loo 2003) (see Table 8.3) can help develop ways in which to tackle project issues or resistance while recording and communicating how they are affecting the overall project status. It can be particularly useful when presenting feedback on project status and in providing a written document to make tracking project management activity transparent.

Project termination phase
This phase should include completing and evaluating the project (Haynes 1989). It is the phase often given least attention. Projects that are never completed successfully are seldom published, precluding the lessons to be learned from practical reasons why projects fail (Tierney 1997). Often teams are so thankful that a project is finished that they forget to adequately debrief and evaluate the accuracy of their preplanning (Shirey 2008). Lessons learned can be applied to future project management efforts (Shirey 2008). Critical evaluation of the example project leads to the creation of a template for the project

Table 8.1 Generic project planning chart

Activity	Accountability	Estimated time	Elapse time	Required resources
1.1	Ward Senior	1 day	1 week	Shelving
1.2	Med Engineer	1 day	7 weeks	Testing equipment
1.4	Project Manager	1 hour	1 week	Information from theatre
1.6	Coagulation Nurse Specialist	1 hour	7 weeks	Funding for printing leaflets
2.1	Project Manager	1 week	7 weeks	One Link nurse for each surgical ward
2.2, 2.3, 2.4	PDNs, Coagulation Nurses, Industry	7 weeks ongoing	0	Deliver training regularly using standard training package
2.5, 2.6, 2.7	Project Manager	1 week	0	Document training intervals based on findings and disseminate standard training package
2.8	Medical Engineering/ Project Manager	7 weeks ongoing	0	Medical Engineering to keep list of those trained; Project Manager to ensure that all trainers are aware of need to keep list of those trained and to forward information to Medical Engineering
3.1	Procurement	1 day	0	Supply Project Manager with costings
3.2, 3.3, 3.4	Project Manager	1 hour	When 3.1 completed	Leadership and negotiation skills

(Adapted from Loo 2003)

Table 8.2 Issues analysis chart

Issue/problem	Impact assessment	Action to be taken
Allocating time for project team to train staff and for staff to attend training	Could be high impact, as we cannot complete project until 50% of staff are trained; medium probability, as we have been progressing well with training so far	Ask industry to provide extra nurse trainers Negotiate with each ward sister the best time to provide training for staff to attend Inform stakeholders if delay in achieving target is anticipated
Funding for disposables on the wards may be declined	Could be low impact, as the disposables would already be attached to the patients when they leave Recovery; low probability, as the consequences of VTE are serious and risk management would validate any extra cost	Determine actual cost implications Negotiate with industry and procurement to get best deal Project manager to use leadership skills to influence budget holders Inform stakeholders if this becomes an issue Rally support from Chief Executive
Staff sickness within Coagulation Team	Could be high impact, as project manager would be redeployed to cover staff sickness; medium probability if related to previous sickness rates	Delegate project tasks if appropriate Draft staff from other areas to cover Coagulation Inform stakeholders immediately if still short-staffed Consider reducing other coagulation services if project deadline is close, or amending task deadlines if they will still complete prior to project deadline Work overtime if agreed by Project Manager and funding or time back agreed by management

Table 8.3 Work progress sheet. Reporting period, 8 October 2008–8 December 2008. Prepared by Project Manager

Project status A brief description of activities completed since last project status report	1. Ward selected and agreed to store IPC 2. *Ad hoc* training continues via industry, Coagulation Nurse Specialists and Project Manager. Two Link Nurses enlisted 3. Literature produced on IPC: checklist, equipment tag, A5 card for safe use of machine, patient information leaflet supplied by Industry passed the Trust Patient Information Leaflet Group 4. Funding for IPC disposables not secured

Issues and actions taken
What problems have arisen during the reporting period and how have they been resolved?
	1.
	  • Led meeting with Equipment Manager, Site Manager and industry to agree on storage area: disagreement on where to store equipment
	  • Users to decide on storage area (Surgical Head of Nursing)
	  • Head of Nursing has advised Ward Senior to arrange shelving
	2.
	  • Training needs to be standardized
	  • List of names of those trained not being kept, Medical Engineering to keep list and Project Manager to inform all trainers to pass on names
	  • Need Link Nurse for each surgical ward
	  • Need to involve PDNs as trainers
	3.
	  • Generic patient information leaflet on VTE RA and TP developed, but awaiting approval from Trust Patient Information Leaflet Group and funding for publishing needs to be sought
	4.
	  • Meeting with industry, procurement, Project Manager and Lead for Thrombosis Committee to get written agreement of contract
	  • Negotiate with budget holder to secure funding
	  • Procurement to provide figures on expenditure for disposables year-on-year

Upcoming milestones Record changes to work plans	1. Shelving to be erected by end of December 2008 2. Trust generic patient information leaflet should be passed for use by end of December 2008

Table 8.4 Project management process and tools template for venous thromboembolism risk assessment and thromboprophylaxis implementation

Project management process	Preferred tools	Useful alternatives
Conceptual phase	SWOT analysis Project description	Situational analysis Issues impact assessment worksheet
Project planning phase	Work breakdown structure (form SMART objectives) Generic project planning chart Issues analysis chart	Gantt chart
Implementation phase	Worksheet progress report	Amend plans as necessary
Project termination phase	Critical evaluation of project management Dissemination of learning gained	Debriefing Structured reflection

(Kindly reproduced by permission of Thrombus, who retain the copyright. All rights reserved.)

management process and tools appropriate for the strategic planning and implementation of VTE risk assessment and thromboprophylaxis (Table 8.4).

A tightly structured approach to project management is not always necessary and may dampen creativity (Tierney 1997). However, due to funding issues in the health sector, reality may require very detailed planning to manage projects to time. Billows (2008) warns that a very detailed breakdown of the WBS can lead to micromanagement and discourages independence of the project team, yet the generic project planning chart (Loo 2003) has a column for accountability, which potentially empowers the project team. Ethical dilemmas therefore present when making decisions on project management issues and, to stand the best chance of success, should take into account the Project Manager's own personal management style and the organizational culture where the change is to be introduced.

Loo (2003) describes project management as a core competency for nurses. As the scope of Clinical Nurse Specialist (CNS) projects becomes more complex, there is a need to use project management tools to help enhance CNS performance (Shirey 2008).

The success of implementation needs to be evaluated through clinical audit. Currently the Department of Health is reviewing the nursing metrics relating to VTE and will advise on ways to evaluate safety, efficacy and compassion or satisfaction with VTE prevention methods.

Balancing the vision with reality – note from the author

Creativity is important to identify novel ways of achieving objectives. Link nurses can provide leadership locally to facilitate education and implementation of thromboprophylaxis. An outline of the Coagulation Link Nurse role is demonstrated in Box 8.7.

I originally enrolled to do 'Advanced Nursing Knowledge' as my next Master's module. However, this would have required learning a new topic. Due to unforeseen sickness within our team, I did not have enough time to learn a new topic, meet the book chapter deadline and deliver on my work project deadline, whereas I could enrol instead on a 'Work Based Learning' (project management) module to increase my chances of achieving my work objective within the time frame set and combine it with a topic relevant to the book chapter, while maintaining my professional development. This is an example of how reorganizing my overall workload using leadership and project management skills facilitated the achievement of meeting several important objectives. This provided a new construct in my knowledge base, and the learning gained through the experience may useful to

---

Box 8.7 Coagulation Link Nurse role

Implementation was assisted by the introduction of coagulation link nurses. These were designated local leaders or champions on each ward who could facilitate the change. They were tasked with various challenges, such as:

- Implement individualized VTE nursing care plan for each patient (see Box 8.1).
- Increasing awareness of the need for 100% VTE risk assessment.
- Training of all staff on IPC/AES and ensuring that adequate literature and tape measures are available.
- Ensuring that thromboprophylaxis products are in stock in their clinical area.
- Development of a specialist/expert knowledge base on VTE risk assessment and thromboprophylaxis and anticoagulation and VTE treatment in relation to their own clinical area.
- Incorporating this role into their appraisals.

others as many clinicians struggle with delivering on deadlines when faced with the challenges within the workplace.

Informing the patient

Patients can be informed in various ways. Opportunities for face-to-face education should be taken during any patient–nurse interactions, ideally during VTE risk assessment consultations. Often time constraints in the work place limit these opportunities, but patients should still be provided with access to further information. Easily accessible patient information leaflets should be stocked on wards and in clinics (see Appendix 2 for an example relating to VTE risk assessment and thromboprophylaxis). Online information is readily available from sites such as NHS Choices, an online service that aims to help patients make choices about their own health, from lifestyle decisions such as exercise through to the practical aspects of accessing NHS services, thereby putting patients in control of their own healthcare. Further information on DVT prevention, diagnosis and treatment can be found at:

http://www.nhs.uk/Conditions/Deep-vein-thrombosis/Pages/Introduction.aspx?url=Pages/what-is-it.aspx

Online information for clinicians is available from Map of Medicine, which can also be accessed through NHS Choices:

(http://healthguides.mapofmedicine.com/choices/map/deep_vein_thrombosis1.html).

The direct links to Map of Medicine allows clinicians throughout the NHS to determine the best treatment options for their patients. Another website, this one designed specifically for clinicians, is:

e-VTE (http://e-lfh.org.uk/projects/vte/team.html)

a web-based education resource designed to help raise awareness and improve understanding of VTE. It concentrates on four areas: epidemiology, methods of thromboprophylaxis, implementation of thromboprophylaxis in hospital, and challenges of thromboprophylaxis implementation in primary care. It has been developed by the Department of Health's VTE Implementation Working Group (IWG) in partnership with e-Learning for Healthcare.

To enable implementation of VTE prevention nationally, the Independent Working Group is setting up a network of VTE Exemplar Centres that have a track record of excellent VTE management in either the NHS or the independent sector. These centres provide practical support to other units by sharing their resources to promote best practice in VTE patient care (www.kingsthrombosiscentre.org.uk).

Conclusion

Minimizing the risk of VTE in hospitalized patients requires that evidence-based VTE risk assessment fits into the local organizational culture. Evidence-based thromboprophylaxis should be available for use, and patients and staff should be educated on how to use it. Strong leadership and project management skills will improve the chances of successful implementation.

References

Amarigiri SV, Lees TA (2003) Elastic compression stockings for prevention of deep vein thrombosis. In *The Cochrane Library*. Wiley, Chichester.

Arcelus JI, Caprini JA, Hoffman KN *et al.* (1995) Modifications of plasma levels of tissue factor pathway inhibitor and endothelial-1 induced by a reverse Trendelenburg position: influence of elastic compression – preliminary results. *Journal of Vascular Surgery* **22**: 568–572.

Benko T, Kalik I, Chetty MN (1999) The physiological effect of graded compression stockings on blood flow in the lower limb: an assessment with colour Doppler ultrasound. *Phlebology* **14**: 17–20.

Billows D (2008) *How many tasks in the WBS?* Available at: http://www.4pm.com/articles/wbs.html

British Standard 7672 (1993) Specification for compression, stiffness and labelling of anti-embolism hosiery. Available at: http://www.standardsdirect.org/standards/standards5/StandardsCatalogue24_view_6804.html

Burns JM (1978) *Leadership*. Harper and Row, New York.

CEP (2008) Available at: http://www.pasa.nhs.uk/PASAWeb/NHSprocurement/CEP/CEPproducts/CEP+catalogue.htm#Buyers%20guide

Chief Nursing Officer (2009) *CNO Bulletin*, February 2009. Available at: http://www.dh.gov.uk/en/Publicationsandstatistics/Bulletins/Chiefnursingofficerbulletin/Browsable/DH_095366

Coleridge Smith PD, Hasty JH, Scurr JH (1991) Deep vein thrombosis: effect of graduated compression stockings on distension of the deep veins of the calf. *British Journal of Surgery* **78**(6): 724–726.

Department of Health (DH) (2007) *Report of the Independent Expert Working Group on the Prevention of Venous Thromboembolism in Hospitalised Patients.* DH, London. Available at: http://www.dh.gov.uk/en/ PublicationsandstatisticspolicyAndGuidance/DH_073944

Department of Health (DH) (2002) *Shifting the Balance of Power: The Next Steps.* DH, London. Available at: http://tinyurl.com/58fh8n

Elliott CG, Dudney TM, Egger M *et al.* (1999) Calf–thigh sequential pneumatic compression compared with plantar venous pneumatic compression to prevent deep-vein thrombosis after non-lower extremity trauma. *Journal of Trauma* **47**: 25–32.

Faghri PD, Pompe Van Meerdervort HF, Glaser RM *et al.* (1997) Electrical stimulation-induced contraction to reduce blood stasis during arthroplasty. *Rehabilitation Engineering* **5**: 62–69.

Geerts WH, Bergqvist D, Pineo GF *et al.* (2008) Prevention of venous thromboembolism. American College of Chest Physicians evidence based clinical practice guidelines, 8th Edition. *Chest* **133**: 381–453S.

Haynes ME (1989) *Project Management: from Idea to Implementation.* Crisp Publications Inc., Menlo Park, CA.

Hartmann JT (1982) Cyclic sequential compression of the lower limb in prevention of DVT. *Journal of Bone and Joint Surgery* **62**: 1059–1062.

Hoppensteadt DA, Jeske W, Fareed J *et al.* (1995) The role of TFPI in the mediation of the antithrombotic actions of heparin and LMWH. *Blood Coagulation and Fibrinolysis* **6**: 57–64S.

Jacobs DG, Piotrowski JJ, Hoppensteadt DA *et al.* (1996) Hemodynamic and fibrinolytic consequences of IPC: preliminary results, *Journal of Trauma, Injury, Infection and Critical Care* **40**: 710–717.

Loo R (2003) Project management: a core competency for professional nurses and nurse managers. *Journal for Nurses in Staff Development* **19**: 187–193.

National Institute for Health and Clinical Excellence (NICE) (2007) *Venous Thromboembolism (Deep Vein Thrombosis and Pulmonary Embolism) in Patients Undergoing Surgery.* London, NICE. Available at: http://guidance.nice.org. uk/CG046

Newton R (2005) *The Project Manager.* Harlow, Pearson Education Ltd.

Nursing and Midwifery Council (NMC) (2008) The code: standards of conduct, performance and ethics for nurses and midwives: Available at: http://www. nmc-uk.org/aArticle.aspx?ArticleID=3056

Pischke-Winn K, Minnick, A (1996) Project management: lessons learned from introducing a multitask environmental worker program. *Journal of Nursing Administration* **26**: 31–38.

Shirey M (2008) Project management tools for leaders and entrepreneurs. *Clinical Nurse Specialist* **22**: 129–131.

Sigel B, Edelstein AL, Savitch L *et al.* (1975) Type of compression for reducing venous stasis. A study of lower extremities during inactive recumbency. *Archives of Surgery* **110**: 171–175.

Scottish Intercollegiate Guidelines Network (SIGN) (2002) *National Clinical Guidelines on Prophylaxis of Venous Thromboembolism.* University of Dundee. Available at: http://www.sign.ac.uk/pdf/sign62.pdf

Tierney A (1997) Planning and managing a research project to time. *Nurse Researcher* **5**: 35–50.

Urbankova J, Quiroz R, Kucher N *et al.* (2005) IPC and DVT prevention. A meta-analysis in post-op patients. *Thrombosis and Haemostasis* **94**: 1181–1185.

Virchow R (1856) Emboli der Lungenarterie. *Arch Path Anat* **10**: 225–228.

Wright S (1996) Unlock the leadership potential. *Nursing Management* **3**: 8–10.

Risk assessment for venous thromboembolism (VTE)

Risk assessment is recommended for all patients on admission to hospital. It is recommended that all patients are periodically reassessed during inpatient stay, as risk may change. Reassessment after at least 48–72 hours is advised.

Step one

Review the patient-related factors shown on the assessment sheet against thrombosis risk (Table A1), ticking each box that applies (more than one box can be ticked). Use the highest category of risk if more than one box is ticked (e.g. if both moderate and high risk are ticked, use guidance for high-risk patients).

Any tick for thrombosis risk should prompt thromboprophylaxis, according to local policy.

The risk factors identified are not exhaustive. Clinicians may consider additional risks in individual patients and offer thromboprophylaxis as appropriate.

Step two

Review the patient-related factors shown against bleeding risk and tick each box that applies (more than one box can be ticked).

Venous Thromboembolism: A Nurses Guide to Prevention and Management   By Ellen Welch
© 2010 John Wiley & Sons, Ltd.

Table A1 Risk assessment for venous thromboembolism (VTE)

	Patient-related	Procedure-related	Tick
Thrombosis risk			
High	Age > 60 years		
	Previous pulmonary embolism or deep vein thrombosis		
	Active cancer		
	Acute or chronic lung disease		
	Acute or chronic inflammatory disease		
	Chronic heart failure		
	Lower limb paralysis (excluding acute stroke)		
	Acute infectious disease, e.g. pneumonia		
	BMI >30 kg/m²		
		Hip or knee replacement	
		Hip fracture	
		Other major orthopaedic surgery	
Moderate		Surgical procedure lasting >30 minutes	
		Plaster cast immobilization of lower limb	
Bleeding risk			
	Haemophilia or other known bleeding disorder		
	Known platelet count <100		
	Acute stroke in previous month (haemorrhagic or ischaemic)		
	Blood pressure >200 systolic or 120 diastolic		
	Severe liver disease (prothrombin time above normal or known varices)		
	Severe renal disease		
	Active bleeding		
	Major bleeding risk, existing anticoagulant therapy or antiplatelet therapy		
		Neurosurgery, spinal surgery or eye surgery	
		Other procedure with high bleeding risk	
		Lumbar puncture/spinal/ epidural in previous 4 hours	

Any tick for bleeding risk should prompt clinical staff to consider whether bleeding risk is sufficient to preclude pharmacological intervention.

Step three

If the form has been filled out correctly and no boxes are ticked, then the patient is at low risk of venous thromboembolism and no intervention is indicated.

Guidance on thromboprophylaxis is available at:

- *Surgical patients.* See *Venous Thromboembolism: Reducing the Risk in Surgical Inpatients.* National Institute for Health and Clinical Excellence: http://www.nice.org.uk/nicemedia/pdf/VTEFullGuide.pdf
- *Medical patients.* See *Report of the Independent Expert Working Group on the Prevention of Venous Thromboembolism in Hospitalised Patients.* Department of Health: http://www.dh.gov.uk/en/Publicationsandstatistics/Publications/PublicationsPolicyAndGuidance/DH_073944
- *Obstetric patients.* The risk assessment is not intended for use in pregnant women. See *Thromboprophylaxis during Pregnancy, Labour and after Vaginal Delivery (37),* January 2004. Royal College of Obstetricians and Gynaecologists: http://www.rcog.org.uk/index.asp?PageID=535 (this document has been authorized by the Department of Health). Gateway Reference No: 10278.

This document has been authorized by the Department of Health

Patient information leaflet on VTE prevention from King's College Hospital NHS Foundation Trust

Who should read this patient guide?

This guide has been written for you if you are being admitted to hospital in the near future. It is intended to help you understand venous blood clots **(called venous thromboembolism or VTE for short)**, which can form in your body after illness or surgery. After reading this guide, you may wish to discuss VTE with your doctor and ask about the best way to reduce the likelihood of this condition.

What is VTE?

VTE is the name given to a deep vein thrombosis **(called DVT for short)** or a pulmonary embolism **(called PE for short).** A DVT is a thrombus (blood clot) that forms in a deep vein, most commonly in your leg or pelvis, and can cause **swelling and pain**. In the longer term, DVT can cause painful, long-term swelling and ulcers. If a clot becomes dislodged and passes through your circulation and reaches your lungs, this is called a PE and can cause **coughing (with blood stained phlegm), chest pain and breathlessness.** VTE diagnosis requires immediate treatment. **If you develop any of these symptoms either in hospital or after discharge, please seek medical advice immediately.**

Venous Thromboembolism: A Nurses Guide to Prevention and Management By Ellen Welch
© 2010 John Wiley & Sons, Ltd.

Is VTE common?

VTE occurs in the general population in about one in 500 people. You will have heard in the news about DVT in people flying for long periods and suffering from 'economy class syndrome', but you are actually much more likely to get VTE if you are going into hospital because of illness or for surgery. About one in eight patients going into hospital because of illness and up to one in two patients admitted to hospital for surgery will develop VTE if no protection is provided.

Who is at risk of VTE?

In addition to admission to hospital, there are other factors which place you at greater risk of VTE. These include a previous VTE, a recent diagnosis of cancer, and certain blood conditions such as clotting disorders. In addition, certain contraceptive and hormone replacement tablets can increase your risk.

Will my risk of VTE be assessed?

The Government recognizes VTE is an important problem in hospitals and has advised doctors and nurses that everyone being admitted to hospital should have a risk assessment completed. Your individual risk for VTE will be assessed by your clinical team. If you are at risk, your doctor or nurse will discuss with you what can be done to reduce your risk and will follow national guidelines and offer you protection against VTE.

What can I do to reduce my risk of VTE?

If your hospital admission has been planned several weeks in advance, there are some precautions which you can take to reduce your risk of VTE:

- Talk to your doctor about your contraceptive or hormone replacement tablets. Your doctor may consider stopping them in the weeks before your operation.
- Avoid travelling for more than three hours in the month before your operation if possible.
- Keep a healthy weight.

When in hospital:

- Keep moving or walking; leg exercises are valuable. You can ask to see a physiotherapist if you would like to learn some leg exercises.
- Ask your doctor or nurse, 'What is being done to reduce my risk of VTE?'
- Drink plenty of fluid to keep hydrated.

In hospital, what will be done to reduce my risk of VTE?

If you are having an operation, ask your anaesthetist to consider which type of anaesthesia is most appropriate for you.

Anti-embolism stockings – if considered appropriate by your doctor, you will be measured and fitted with thigh-length stockings depending on your leg measurements. You should be shown how to wear them and advised to report any new symptoms in your feet or legs when wearing them to a doctor. These will reduce your risk of VTE.

The clinical team may ask you to wear a special *inflatable sleeve or cuff around your legs* while you are in bed. This will inflate automatically and provide pressure at regular intervals, increasing blood flow out of your legs. If they have been removed for more than three hours they should not be reapplied, unless agreed by a doctor.

Finally, your doctor might consider that you should take an *anticoagulant injection or tablet*, which reduces the chance of your blood clotting and stop DVT from forming. The drug normally prescribed at King's College Hospital is heparin, which is given by injection. There are new drugs becoming available in tablet form, which may be offered to you.

To be effective, these methods of prevention must be fitted, used and administered correctly, so if you have any questions or concerns, please ask your doctor for advice.

What happens after I have been discharged from hospital?

Anti-embolism stockings should be worn from admission until you return to your usual level of mobility. If you have been advised to continue anticoagulation medicine at home and you need help with administration of injections or tablets, please ask your nurse before discharge. **If you develop any signs or symptoms of VTE at home, then seek medical advice immediately, either from your GP (home doctor) or your nearest hospital emergency department.**

Where can I find out more?

Please ask your doctor or nurse for more information. Alternatively, the NHS Choices website provides patient information on VTE at: www.nhs.uk

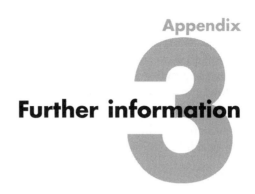

Further information

National and international guidelines

Prophylaxis of Venous Thromboembolism. Scottish Intercollegiate Guidelines Network, October 2002. Available at: www.sign.ac.uk/guidelines/fulltext/62/

The British Thoracic Society Guidelines for the Management of Suspected Acute Pulmonary Embolism. British Thoracic Society Standards of Care Committee Pulmonary Embolism Guideline Development Group. Available at: http://thorax.bmj.com/cgi/content/extract/58/6/470

Thromboprophylaxis during Pregnancy, Labour and after Vaginal Delivery (Guideline No. 37) and *Venous Thromboembolism and Hormonal Contraception Delivery* (Guideline No. 40). Royal College of Obstetrics and Gynaecology, January 2004. Available at: www.rcog.org.uk

Thromboembolic Disease in Pregnancy and the Puerperium: Acute Management (Green-top Guideline No. 28). Royal College of Obstetrics and Gynaecology, February 2007. Available at: www.rcog.org.uk

The Diagnosis of DVT in Symptomatic Outpatients. British Committee for Standards in Haematology, January 2004. Available at: www.bcshguidelines.com/pdf/dvt_220506.pdf

Procedures for the Outpatient Management of Patients with Deep Venous Thrombosis. British Committee for Standards in Haematology, January 2004. Available at: www.bcshguidelines.com/pdf/dvt_220506.pdf

Venous Thromboembolism: A Nurses Guide to Prevention and Management   By Ellen Welch
© 2010 John Wiley & Sons, Ltd.

The Prevention of Venous Thromboembolism in Hospitalised Patients (Second Report of Session 2004–2005). The Department of Health, May 2005. Available at: www.dh.gov.uk/en/Publicationsandstatistics/Publications/PublicationsPolicyAndGuidance/DH_4116284

Guidelines on the Use and Monitoring of Heparin. British Committee for Standard in Haematology, April 2006. Available at: www.bcshguidelines.com/pdf/heparin_220506.pdf

Prevention and Treatment of Venous Thromboembolism (International Consensus Statement). The International Union of Angiology, October 2006. Available at: www.minervamedica.it/en/journals/international-angiology/article.php?cod=R34Y2006N02A0101

Reducing the Risk of Venous Thromboembolism in Inpatients Undergoing Surgery. The National Institute for Health and Clinical Excellence CG046, April 2007. Available at: www.nice.org.uk/CG46

Report of the Independent Expert Working Group on the Prevention of Venous Thromboembolism in Hospitalised Patients. Department of Health, April 2007. Available at: www.dh.gov.uk/en/Publichealth/Healthprotection/Bloodsafety/VenousThromboembolismVTE/DH_073963

Recommendations for Venous Thromboembolism Prophylaxis and Treatment in Patients with Cancer. The American Society of Clinical Oncology Guideline, December 2007. Available at: http://jco.ascopubs.org/cgi/content/short/25/34/5490

The 8th American College of Chest Physicians Conference on Antithrombotic and Thrombolytic Therapy, June 2008:
    Prevention of Venous Thromboembolism
    Antithrombotic Therapy for Venous Thromboembolic Disease
    Antithrombotic Therapy in Children
    Pharmacology and Management of the Vitamin K Antagonists
    Hemorrhagic complications of Anticoagulant and Thrombolytic Treatment
Available at: www.chestnet.org/education/guidelines/currentGuidelines.php

Useful websites

Websites which provide information and advice about venous thromboembolism:

Anticoagulation Europe. Available at: www.anticoagulationeurope. org
Charity committed to the prevention of thrombosis

Clotcare. Available at: www.clotcare.com
US charitable organization with an editorial board of experts in anticoagulation; provides up to date information for both patients and professionals

Department of Health advice on travel related DVT. Available at: www.dh.gov.uk/en/Publichealth/Healthprotection/Bloodsafety/DVT/DH_4123480

Kings Thrombosis Centre. Available at: www.kingsthrombosiscentre. org.uk
The first NHS exemplar centre. Website provides resources on the prevention and treatment of VTE

Lifeblood – The Thrombosis Charity. Available at: www.thrombosis-charity.org.uk
UK charity dedicated to educating patients and professionals on all aspects of thrombosis

National Centre for Anticoagulation Training. Available at: www. anticoagulation.org.uk
Accredited courses for health care professionals involved in anticoagulation management

National Institute for Health and Clinical Excellence. Available at: www.nice.org.uk
Organization responsible for providing national guidance. Guidelines on the prevention of VTE in hospitalized medical patients expected to be published soon

North American Thrombosis Forum. Available at: www.natfonline. org
Multi-disciplinary organization formed to improve patient care through the advancement of thrombosis education

Thrombosis Clinic. Available at: www.thrombosisclinic.com
A continuing medical education resource for healthcare professionals on all aspects of VTE

Thrombosis Research Institute. Available at: www.tri-london.ac.uk
Internationally renowned centre for pioneering research in thrombosis

Venous Thromboembolism Registry (VERITY). Available at: www.verityonline.co.uk
National registry for patients with VTE

VTE Exemplar Centres. Available at: www.kingsthrombosiscentre.org.uk/exemplarcCentres.html
UK hospitals with an existing track record of excellent VTE management who provide practical support to other units by sharing their resources online

Wounds UK. Available at: www.wounds-uk.com
Education in wound management

Glossary

Activated partial thromboplastin time (aPPT)   Blood test carried out to monitor heparin therapy. It measures the time in seconds taken for clotting to occur compared to a 'control' sample of normal blood. If the test sample takes longer than the control, it indicates decreased clotting function in the intrinsic pathway.

Albumin   A plasma protein produced mainly in the liver. Maintains the osmotic pressure between body compartments and acts as a transport protein by binding to several substances.

Alopecia   Hair loss.

Anticoagulant   Substance that prevents the blood from clotting.

Anti-embolism stockings (AES)   Also referred to as graduated compression stockings (GCS); elastic stockings that provide graduated compression for the prevention of VTE.

Anti-factor Xa   The blood test ordered to monitor heparin/LMWH therapy. The only test that works for monitoring LMWH.

Antiphospholipid syndrome   A disorder of coagulation characterized by recurrent venous or arterial thrombosis and/or fetal losses. Occurs due to autoimmune production of antibodies against phospholipid, cardiolipin and β2 glycoprotein 1.

Antithrombin   An inhibitor of thrombin and activated factor X.

Venous Thromboembolism: A Nurses Guide to Prevention and Management   By Ellen Welch
© 2010 John Wiley & Sons, Ltd.

Arterial thrombosis A blood clot within an artery responsible for peripheral vascular disease, heart attacks and embolic strokes.

Atelectasis The collapse of part of the lung usually caused by blockage to the small airways.

Atrial septal defect A congenital heart defect characterized by a hole in the wall (the septum) that separates the right and left atria.

Bifurcation A division into two or more branches.

Bioavailability The degree to which a substance (such as a drug) becomes available for activity in the target tissue after administration.

Bleeding disorder The term used to describe the range of conditions that present with prolonged bleeding.

Blood gas partial pressures Blood gas partial pressures are reported by some laboratories in kiloPascals (kPa) and by others in millimetres of mercury (mmHg). Here is a guide to convert between the two:

$1\,kPA = 7.5\,mmHg$
$1\,mmHg = 0.133\,kPa$

Normal arterial blood gas (ABG) values:

Arterial pO_2	11.2–13.9 kPa	84–104 mmHg
Arterial pCO_2	4.7–6.1 kPa	35–45 mmHg
Arterial pH	7.35–7.45	35–45 nmol l^{-1} of H$^+$
Arterial [HCO_3^-]		22–26 mmol l^{-1}

Capillary Smallest blood vessels, where blood and interstitial fluid exchange material.

Chronic venous insufficiency (CVI) Impaired venous return, sometimes causing lower extremity discomfort, oedema and skin changes. Postphlebitic (post-thrombotic) syndrome is symptomatic chronic venous insufficiency after DVT.

Clot Another term for 'thrombus'. Describes a jelly-like substance that plugs a hole in a blood vessel to stop blood from leaking out.

Coagulation Process of clot formation. The protein-based clotting factors work together to convert blood from liquid to a semi-fluid clot consistency.

Coagulant Substance that plays a role in blood clotting.

Coagulation cascade The sequence of interactions between the clotting factors in blood which culminates in the production of fibrin.

Coagulation factors   Substances in the blood that undergo chemical reactions which result in blood clotting.

Cofactors   Substances that work alongside factors in the coagulation cascade to promote the process.

Collateral circulation   Secondary route the blood takes to circulate, aside from the main anatomical route.

Common pathway   The pathway resulting from the merging of the extrinsic and intrinsic pathways of the coagulation cascade – the final steps before a clot is formed.

Concentrates   Fractionated freeze-dried preparations of individual clotting factors or groups of factors which provide rapid treatment for bleeding patients.

Creatinine clearance   A test of renal function. Creatinine is a substance formed during metabolism and filtered out of the blood by the kidneys. Levels are elevated in renal failure.

Cryoprecipitate   The solid material that forms when plasma is slowly thawed.

Cyanotic   A blue discoloration of the skin due to a lack of oxygen in the blood.

Cytoplasm   The contents of a cell other than the nucleus and the cell wall.

D-dimer   A breakdown product of fibrin.

Deep vein thrombosis (DVT)   Venous thrombosis that occurs in the 'deep veins' of the legs, thighs or pelvis. Asymptomatic DVT is defined as DVT detected by screening using techniques such as ultrasound or ascending venography, while symptomatic DVT presents with leg pain or swelling resulting from occlusion of a major vein.

Depolymerization   The conversion of a compound into one of a smaller molecular weight and different physical properties.

Disseminated intravascular coagulation (DIC)   A serious coagulopathy resulting from the uncontrolled activation of clotting factors and fibrinolytic enzymes in response to disease or injury, resulting in tissue necrosis and bleeding.

Dorsiflexion   Upward movement of the feet or toes.

Dysproteinaemia   An abnormality in the protein content of blood.

ELISA (enzyme-linked immunosorbent assay) Biochemical technique used to detect the presence of an antibody or an antigen in a sample using a measurable enzyme.

Endothelial cells The cells that line the interior surface of blood vessels.

Enzyme A protein capable of catalysing (accelerating) a biological reaction.

Enzyme cofactors Some enzymes require non-protein molecules to bind to them to enable full activity. These molecules are known as cofactors.

Enzyme precursors A chemical that is transformed into another compound in the course of a chemical reaction.

Epistaxis Nose bleed.

Erythrocyte Red blood cell which transports oxygen from the lungs to the tissues.

Extracorporeal Outside or unrelated to the body.

Extrinsic pathway One of the three pathways of the coagulation cascade activated by exposure of blood to tissue factor, circulating factor VII, calcium and phospholipid.

Factor deficiencies The term to describe a number of conditions which manifest as an abnormality of proteins involved in blood clotting.

Factor V Leiden A common inherited genetic disorder of coagulation resulting in an increased tendency to clot and therefore an increased risk of VTE.

Fascia A sheet of fibrous connective tissue below the skin that separates or binds together muscles and organs.

Foramen ovale An opening in the septum between the right and left atria of the heart, present in the fetus but usually closing soon after birth.

Fresh frozen plasma (FFP) Human plasma separated from blood cells and platelets within hours of donation and frozen at −30 °C. It contains all the clotting factors but at a very low concentration to volume.

Fibrin Threadlike protein found in the blood which meshes together to form the foundation for a clot.

Fibrinolytic system The system responsible for the breakdown of fibrin. Balances the clotting activity of blood.

Haemarthrosis   Bleeding into a joint space (usually causing the joint capsule to swell).

Haematemesis   Vomiting of blood due to internal bleeding.

Haematoma   Accumulation of blood in the soft tissues.

Haemophilia   The name given to a range of disorders which manifest as prolonged bleeding. Haemophilia A (classical haemophilia) is due to a factor VIII deficiency. Haemophilia B (Christmas disease) results from a deficiency of factor IX. Haemophilia C is sometimes used to describe a deficiency of factor XI.

Haemorrhage   Bleeding with loss of large quantities of blood.

Haemostasis   The stopping of bleeding.

Hyperemesis gravidarum   Extreme, persistent nausea and vomiting during pregnancy that can lead to dehydration and ketosis.

Hyperkalaemia   High potassium.

Hypertension   High blood pressure.

Hypoaldosteronism   A deficiency of aldosterone in the body.

Hypovolaemia   Low circulating blood volume.

Iatrogenic   Caused by medical personnel or medical procedures.

Idiopathic   Of unknown cause.

IgG (immunoglobulin G)   The most abundant antibody. Triggers the complement system required for the immune response.

IgM (immunoglobulin M)   The largest antibody and the first produced when the body is challenged by antigens. Triggers the production of IgG.

Inflammation   The term used to describe congestion of the blood vessels and surrounding tissues, manifested by redness, swelling, heat and pain.

International Normalised ratio (INR)   A comparative rating of a patient's prothrombin time (PT), measured against international standards, for monitoring the effects of warfarin.

Intra-articular haemorrhage   Bleeding into a joint.

Intramuscular haemorrhage   Bleeding into a muscle.

Intravenous   Inside a vein – 'i.v.' injections are given into the vein.

Intrinsic pathway   One of the three pathways of the coagulation cascade activated when blood comes into contact with negatively charged surface, exposed as a result of tissue damage.

Ionizing radiation   High-energy radiation (such as that produced by X-rays) that is capable of damaging living tissue at a molecular level.

Latex agglutination test   A method of detecting the presence of an antibody in which antigen is adsorbed onto latex particles, which then clump in the presence of a specific antibody.

Lipodermatosclerosis   Skin change of lower legs from inflammation of subcutaneous fat due to venous insufficiency, characterized by hardened skin with increased pigmentation, swelling and erythema.

Morbidity   The condition of being ill. In statistics it describes the rate at which illness occurs in a particular population.

Mortality   The death rate.

Negative predictive value   The probability that a patient with a negative test result is really free from the condition for which the test was conducted.

Nomogram   A graphical representation of a numerical relationship, used in practice as tools to determine, for example, appropriate medication doses based on INR results.

Osteoblasts   Cells in the body that build new bone tissue.

Osteoclasts   Bone cells that break down and remove bone tissue.

Osteopenia   A reduction in bone mass below normal levels, usually caused by a lower rate of bone formation compared to bone destruction. A risk factor for the development of osteoporosis.

Osteoporosis   A reduction in both bone mass and bone mineral density, resulting in fragile bones which break easily.

Pentasaccharide   A carbohydrate which is made up of five 'monosaccharides' or simple sugar residues.

Pharmacokinetics   The branch of pharmacology that explores what the body does to a drug, looking at mechanisms of absorption and distribution, the rate at which drug action begins, the duration of effect, chemical changes that occur in the body and the routes of excretion. In contrast, *pharmacodynamics* looks at what the drug does to the body.

Pitting oedema   Fluid in the subcutaneous tissues that retains the indentation caused by pressure – usually present in the extremities.

Plasma   The liquid portion of blood, which contains many proteins including clotting factors, immunoglobulins and albumin.

Plasmin   An enzyme that breaks down fibrin.

Platelets   Sticky, plate-shaped components of blood, which assist in clotting by sticking to the vessel wall around injury sites.

Polycythaemia   Condition caused by an abnormally large number of red blood cells in the circulation.

Positive predictive value   The probability that a patient with a positive test result really does have the condition for which the test was conducted.

Post-thrombotic (postphlebitic) leg syndrome   Chronic pain, swelling, dermatitis and occasional ulceration of the skin, occurring as a consequence of previous destruction of leg vein valves by DVT. Leg ulcers are found in 2–10% of patients 10 years after their first symptomatic DVT, and about 0.2% of the general population have venous ulcers (SIGN 2002).

Prophylaxis   A measure taken for the prevention of disease.

Prothrombin complex concentrates (PCC)   Freeze-dried powder preparations of coagulation factors II, IX, X and VII.

Proton   A small positively charged particle found in the nucleus of all atoms.

Pseudopodia   Temporary protrusions of the cytoplasm of a cell that aid with locomotion or food uptake.

PT (prothrombin time)   Blood test that measures the time taken for clot formation after thromboplastin and calcium is added to a sample of plasma. Tests the integrity of the intrinsic pathway of the coagulation cascade.

Puerperium   The approximately 6 week period lasting from childbirth until the return of normal uterine size.

Pulmonary embolism (PE)   A blood clot that breaks off from the deep veins and travels round the circulation to block the pulmonary arteries. Most deaths arising from DVT are caused by PE. A 'massive' PE is one so severe as to cause circulatory collapse.

Pulmonary thromboendarterectomy   Operative procedure that removes thrombi from the pulmonary circulation.

Purpura fulminans Rare vascular disorder resulting from hereditary or acquired protein C deficiency, protein S deficiency, activated protein C resistance or disseminated intravascular coagulation. Manifests as haemorrhagic skin necrosis due to dermal vascular thrombosis and is associated with fever, shock and multiorgan failure.

Qualitative Associated with the subjective quality of data, in contrast to *quantitative* which pertains to amounts.

Quantitative Associated with the measurement of numerical data.

Recombinant Material produced by genetic engineering.

SATS Refers to the percentage of haemaglobin binding sites in the blood occupied by (or saturated by) oxygen. In practice, this is measured using pulse oximetry, a non-invasive device which, when placed on a digit, monitors the light absorption of haemoglobin to give an indication of oxygen saturation. Arterial blood gas analysis (ABG) offers more reliable results but is invasive. Normal range, 95–100%.

Sensitivity The 'sensitivity' of a test refers to the probability that the test is positive when given to a group of patients with the disease. A high sensitivity means that a negative test can rule out the disease.

Serum Plasma with the clotting factors removed.

Specificity The probability that the test will be negative among patients who do not have the disease. A high specificity means that a positive test can rule in the disease.

Subcutaneous 'Under the skin', usually used in the context of s.c. injections – meaning injections into the fatty tissue beneath the skin.

Tachycardia A heart rate >100 beats per minute.

Tachypnoea A respiratory rate >20 breaths per minute.

Telangiectasia Chronic dilatation of capillaries at the surface of the skin, causing dark red blotches.

Thrombocytopenia Abnormally low concentration of platelets in the blood. May result in bleeding into the skin or spontaneous bruising.

Thrombophlebitis Many words have been used throughout history to describe venous thrombosis, so there is often confusion when reading the literature as to what the author is describing. The accepted solution today is to reserve the term 'deep vein thrombosis' for thrombosis in the deep veins, and to use the term 'thrombophlebitis' for superficial thrombosis. 'Thrombophlebitis' is therefore a combination of thrombosis and phlebitis in a superficial vein.

Thromboprophylaxis   A measure taken to prevent thrombosis.

Varicose eczema   Also known as 'stasis dermatitis'. Irritable, sensitive skin secondary to venous insufficiency.

Venous ectasia   Venous expansion/dilatation.

Venous thromboembolism (VTE)   The blocking of a blood vessel by a clot dislodged from its site of origin. It includes both DVT and PE.

Vitamin K antagonists   Anticoagulants such as warfarin that reduce the amount of vitamin K available for the activation of coagulation factors II, VII, IX and X.

Von Willebrand factor   A glycoprotein in blood, involved in haemostasis.

Index

Venous Thromboembolism: A Nurses Guide to Prevention and Management   By Ellen Welch
© 2010 John Wiley & Sons, Ltd.